Parey

ATLAS OF RADIOGRAPHIC ANATOMY OF THE CAT

Part 2 of "ATLAS OF RADIOGRAPHIC ANATOMY OF THE DOG AND CAT"

founded by

Dr. Dr. h. c. H. Schebitz †
Univ.-Professor
former Head of the Clinic of Veterinary Surgery
Ludwig-Maximilians-Universität
Munich

Dr. H. Wilkens
Univ.-Professor
former Head of the Institute of Anatomy
Tierärztliche Hochschule
Hanover

1st new edition

by

Dr. H. Waibl
Univ.-Professor
Head of the Institute of Anatomy
Tierärztliche Hochschule
Hanover

Dr. E. Mayrhofer
Univ.-Professor
Head of the Clinic of Radiology
Veterinärmedizinische Universität
Vienna

Dr. U. Matis
Univ.-Professor
Head of the Clinic of Veterinary Surgery
Ludwig-Maximilians-Universität
Munich

Dr. L. Brunnberg
Univ.-Professor
Head of the Clinic and Policlinic of Small Animals
Freie Universität
Berlin

Dr. R. Köstlin
Univ.-Professor
Clinic of Veterinary Surgery
Ludwig-Maximilians-Universität
Munich

English Supervision by
Dr. J. E. Smallwood
Professor of Anatomy
North Carolina State University
Raleigh, NC, USA

With 50 Radiographs, 61 Colored Radiographic Sketches, 51 Positioning Drawings, and 4 Tables

Parey Verlag · Stuttgart

Atlas der Röntgenanatomie der Katze

Teil 2 des „Atlas der Röntgenanatomie von Hund und Katze"

begründet von

Dr. Dr. h. c. H. Schebitz †
Univ.-Professor
ehem. Vorstand der Chirurgischen Tierklinik
Ludwig-Maximilians-Universität
München

Dr. H. Wilkens
Univ.-Professor
ehem. Direktor des Anatomischen Instituts
Tierärztliche Hochschule
Hannover

---

1. Neuauflage

von

Dr. H. Waibl
Univ.-Professor
Direktor des Anatomischen Instituts
Tierärztliche Hochschule
Hannover

Dr. E. Mayrhofer
Univ.-Professor
Vorstand der Klinik für Röntgenologie
Veterinärmedizinische Universität
Wien

Dr. U. Matis
Univ.-Professor
Vorstand der Chirurgischen Tierklinik
Ludwig-Maximilians-Universität
München

Dr. L. Brunnberg
Univ.-Professor
Direktor der Klinik und Poliklinik für kleine Haustiere
Freie Universität
Berlin

Dr. R. Köstlin
Univ.-Professor
Chirurgische Tierklinik
Ludwig-Maximilians-Universität
München

Mit 50 Röntgenbildern, 61 farbigen Röntgenskizzen, 51 Lagerungsskizzen sowie 4 Tabellen

Parey Verlag • Stuttgart

Bibliografische Information
Der Deutschen Bibliothek

Die Deutsche Bibliothek verzeichnet diese Publikation in der Deutschen Nationalbibliographie; detaillierte bibliografische Daten sind im Internet über http://dnb.ddb.de abrufbar.

Anschrift des Herausgebers/Editor's address:
Prof. Dr. Helmut Waibl
Direktor des Anatomischen Instituts
Tierärztliche Hochschule Hannover
Bischofsholer Damm 15
30173 Hannover
Germany

© 2004 Parey Verlag in
MVS Medizinverlage Stuttgart GmbH & Co. KG
Oswald-Hesse-Str. 50, D-70469 Stuttgart

Unsere Homepage: www.parey.de

Printed in Germany

Zeichnungen/Drawings: Anatomisches Institut, Tierärztliche Hochschule Hannover
Umschlaggestaltung/Cover design: Thieme Verlagsgruppe
Umschlaggrafik/Cover graphic: Martina Berge, Erbach
Satz und Repro/Production and set by: XYZ-Satzstudio, Naumburg
Druck/Printed by: Jütte-Messedruck Leipzig
Bindung/Binding: Kunst- und Verlagsbuchbinderei Leipzig

ISBN 3-8304-4100-2

Wichtiger Hinweis:
Wie jede Wissenschaft ist die Veterinärmedizin ständigen Entwicklungen unterworfen. Forschung und klinische Erfahrung erweitern unsere Kenntnisse, insbesondere was Behandlung und medikamentöse Therapie anbelangen. Soweit in diesem Werk eine Dosierung oder eine Applikation erwähnt wird, darf der Leser zwar darauf vertrauen, dass Autoren, Herausgeber und Verlag große Sorgfalt darauf verwandt haben, dass diese Angabe dem **Wissensstand bei Fertigstellung des Werkes entspricht.**

Für Angaben über Dosierungsanweisungen und Applikationsformen kann vom Verlag jedoch keine Gewähr übernommen werden. **Jeder Benutzer ist angehalten,** durch sorgfältige Prüfung der Beipackzettel der verwendeten Präparate – gegebenenfalls nach Konsultation eines Spezialisten – festzustellen, ob die dort gegebene Empfehlung für Dosierungen oder die Beachtung von Kontraindikationen gegenüber der Angabe in diesem Buch abweicht. Eine solche Prüfung ist besonders wichtig bei selten verwendeten Präparaten oder solchen, die neu auf den Markt gebracht worden sind. Vor der Anwendung bei Tieren, die der Lebensmittelgewinnung dienen, ist auf die in den einzelnen deutschsprachigen Ländern unterschiedlichen Zulassungs- und Anwendungsbeschränkungen zu achten. **Jede Dosierung oder Applikation erfolgt auf eigene Gefahr des Benutzers.** Autoren und Verlag appellieren an jeden Benutzer, ihm etwa auffallende Ungenauigkeiten dem Verlag mitzuteilen.

Geschützte Warennamen (Warenzeichen®) werden **nicht immer** besonders kenntlich gemacht. Aus dem Fehlen eines solchen Hinweises kann also nicht geschlossen werden, dass es sich um einen freien Warennamen handelt.

Das Werk, einschließlich aller seiner Teile, ist urheberrechtlich geschützt. Jede Verwendung ist ohne Zustimmung des Verlages außerhalb der engen Grenzen des Urheberrechtsgesetzes unzulässig und strafbar. Das gilt insbesondere für Vervielfältigungen, Übersetzungen, Mikroverfilmungen oder die Einspeicherung und Verarbeitung in elektronischen Systemen.

Important note:
Medicine is an ever-changing science undergoing continual development. Research and clinical experience are continually expanding our knowledge, in particular our knowledge of proper treatment and drug therapy. Insofar as this book mentions any dosage or application, readers may rest assured that the authors, editors, and publishers have made every effort to ensure that such references are in accordance with **the state of knowledge at the time of production of the book.**

Nevertheless, this does not involve, imply, or express any guarantee or responsibility on the part of the publishers in respect to any dosage instructions and forms of applications stated in the book. **Every user is requested to examine carefully** the manufacturers' leaflets accompanying each drug and to check, if necessary in consultation with a physician or specialist, whether the dosage schedules mentioned therein or the contraindications stated by the manufacturers differ from the statements made in the present book. Such examination is particularly important with drugs that are either rarely used or have been newly released on the market. Every dosage schedule or every form of application used is entirely at the user's own risk and responsibility. The authors and publishers request every user to report to the publishers any discrepancies or inaccuracies noticed.

Some of the product names, patents, and registered designs referred to in this book are in fact registered trademarks or proprietary names even though specific reference to this fact is not always made in the text. Therefore, the appearance of a name without designation as proprietary is not to be construed as a representation by the publisher that it is in the public domain.

This book, including all parts thereof, is legally protected by copyright. Any use, exploitation, or commercialization outside the narrow limits set by copyright legislation, without the publisher's consent, is illegal and liable to prosecution. This applies in particular to photostat reproduction, copying, mimeographing, preparation of microfilms, and electronic data processing and storage.

Inhalt

Vorwort zur 1. Neuauflage 9

Einführung 11

Allgemeines zur Lagerung
(H. Waibl, E. Mayrhofer) 12

Hinweise für die Belichtung von Röntgenaufnahmen
(E. Mayrhofer) 14

1 Kopf (H. Waibl, R. Köstlin)

1.1 **Kopf, latero-lateral**
(Kopfknochen, Schädelhöhle) 16
1.2 **Kopf, ventro-dorsal**
(symmetrische Übersicht) 18
1.3 **Kopf, dorso-ventral**
(Kopfknochen, Schädelhöhle) 20
1.4 **Oberkiefer, ventro-dorsal**
(Schrägprojektion, bei geöffneter Mundhöhle) 22
1.5 **Oberkiefer, dorso-ventral**
(Oberkieferzähne, Nasenhöhle) 24
1.6 **Oberkiefer, medio-lateral**
(Schrägprojektion, Oberkiefer, einseitig) 26
1.7 **Unterkiefer, medio-lateral**
(Schrägprojektion, Unterkiefer, einseitig) 27
1.8 **Bulla tympanica, ventro-dorsal**
(Bulla tympanica, symmetrisch) 28

2 Wirbelsäule (H. Waibl, E. Mayrhofer)

2.1 **Halswirbelsäule, latero-lateral**
(gestreckte Halswirbelsäule) 30
2.2 **1. und 2. Halswirbel, rostro-kaudal,** bei geöffneter Mundhöhle
(Atlas, Axis, Dens) 32
2.3. **Halswirbelsäule, ventro-dorsal**
(symmetrische Halswirbelsäule) 34

Allgemeines zur Myelographie (E. Mayrhofer) 36

2.4 **Myelographie, Brust-Lenden-Wirbelsäule, latero-lateral** 38
2.5 **Myelographie, Brust-Lenden-Wirbelsäule, ventro-dorsal** 40

3 Schultergliedmaße (H. Waibl, L. Brunnberg)

3.1 **Schultergelenk, medio-lateral**
(Schultergelenk ohne Überlagerung) 42
3.2 **Schultergelenk, kaudo-kranial**
(Gelenkflächen, sagittal) 43
3.3 **Oberarm, medio-lateral**
(mit Schulter- und Ellbogengelenk) 44
3.4 **Oberarm, kaudo-kranial**
(mit Schulter- und Ellbogengelenk) 45
3.5 **Ellbogengelenk, medio-lateral**
(Condylus, Olekranon, Caput radii, Processus coronoideus) 46
3.6 **Ellbogengelenk, kranio-kaudal**
(Condylus humeri, Gelenkspalt) 47
3.7 **Unterarm, medio-lateral**
(mit Ellbogen- und Karpalgelenk) 48
3.8 **Unterarm, kranio-kaudal**
(mit Ellbogen- und Karpalgelenk) 49
3.9 **Vorderfuß, medio-lateral**
(Karpalgelenk, Mittelfußknochen und Zehen, seitlich) 50
3.10 **Vorderfuß, dorso-palmar**
(Karpalgelenk, Mittelfußknochen und Zehen) 51

Postnatale Entwicklung

Tabelle 3.1 53
3.11 **Schultergelenk, medio-lateral**
(Epi- und Apophyse) 54
3.12 **Schultergelenk, kaudo-kranial**
(Epi- und Apophyse) 54
3.13 **Ellbogengelenk, medio-lateral**
(Epi- und Apophysen) 55
3.14 **Ellbogengelenk, kranio-kaudal**
(Epi- und Apophysen) 55
3.15 **Karpalgelenk, medio-lateral**
(Epiphysen) 56
3.16 **Vorderfuß, dorso-palmar**
(Epiphysen, Sesambeine) 56

4 Beckengliedmaße (H. Waibl, U. Matis, R. Köstlin)

4.1 **Becken, latero-lateral**
(Übersicht) 58
4.2 **Becken, latero-lateral,**
(Schrägprojektion, getrennte Darstellung beider Beckenhälften) 60
4.3 **Becken, ventro-dorsal**
(symmetrische Beckenübersicht) 62
4.4 **Becken, ventro-dorsal**
(einseitige Darstellung des Iliosakralgelenkes) 64
4.5 **Oberschenkel, medio-lateral**
(mit Hüft- und Kniegelenk) 66
4.6 **Oberschenkel, kranio-kaudal**
(mit Hüft- und Kniegelenk) 67
4.7 **Kniegelenk, medio-lateral**
(mit Sesambeinen) 68
4.8 **Kniegelenk, kranio-kaudal**
(mit Sesambeinen) 69
4.9 **Unterschenkel, medio-lateral**
(mit Knie- und Tarsalgelenk) 70
4.10 **Unterschenkel, kranio-kaudal**
(mit Knie- und Tarsalgelenk) 71
4.11 **Hinterfuß, medio-lateral**
(mit Tarsalgelenketagen) 72
4.12 **Hinterfuß, dorso-plantar**
(mit gelenknahen Abschnitten von Tibia und Fibula) 74

Postnatale Entwicklung

Tabelle 4.1 77
4.13 **Hüftgelenk, ventro-dorsal**
(Hüftbein, Epi- und Apophysen) 78
4.14 **Kniegelenk, medio-lateral**
(Epi- und Apophysen, Sesambeine) 79
4.15 **Kniegelenk, kranio-kaudal**
(Epi- und Apophysen, Sesambeine) 79
4.16 **Tarsalgelenk, medio-lateral**
(Epi- und Apophysen) 80
4.17 **Hinterfuß, dorso-plantar**
(Epi- und Apophysen, Sesambeine) 80

5 Thorax (H. Waibl, E. Mayrhofer)

5.1 **Thorax, latero-lateral**
(Brustorgane) 82
5.2 **Thorax, ventro-dorsal**
(Brustorgane) 84
5.3 **Angiokardiographie, latero-lateral**
(Endphase der Systole, venöse Seite) 86
5.4 **Angiokardiographie, latero-lateral**
(Diastole, arterielle Seite) 88

6 Abdomen (H. Waibl, E. Mayrhofer)

6.1 **Abdomen, latero-lateral**
(Übersichtsaufnahme) 90
6.2 **Abdomen, ventro-dorsal**
(Übersichtsaufnahme) 92

Ösophaguskontrolle, Magen-Darm-Kontrastuntersuchung
(E. Mayrhofer) 94

6.3	**Kontrast, Magen, Dünndarm, latero-lateral** (Magenwand, Duodenum) 96
6.4	**Kontrast, Magen, Dünndarm, ventro-dorsal** (Magenwand, Pylorus, Duodenum) 98
6.5	**Kontrast, Darm, latero-lateral** (Magen, Dickdarm) 100
6.6	**Kontrast, Dickdarm, ventro-dorsal** (Übersichtsaufnahme, Dickdarm) 102
6.7	**Cholezystographie, Gallenblase, latero-lateral** (Übersichtsaufnahme) 104
6.8	**Cholezystographie, Gallenblase, ventro-dorsal** (Übersichtsaufnahme) 106

Allgemeines zur Ausscheidungsurographie (Pyelozystographie)
(E. Mayrhofer) 108

6.9	**Pyelographie, latero-lateral** (Nierenbecken, Harnleiter) 110
6.10	**Pyelographie, ventro-dorsal** (Nierenbecken, Harnleiter) 112
6.11	**Zystographie, latero-lateral** (Negativ- und Positiv-Kontrast, Harnblase) 114

7 Literatur 117

Contents

Preface to the 1st new edition 9

Introduction 11

General remarks on positioning
(H. WAIBL, E. MAYRHOFER) 13

Comments on the exposure of x-ray images
(E. MAYRHOFER) 15

1 Head (H. WAIBL, R. KÖSTLIN)

1.1 **Head, latero-lateral**
(cranial bones, cranial cavity) 16
1.2 **Head, ventro-dorsal**
(symmetric survey radiograph) 18
1.3 **Head, dorso-ventral**
(cranial bones, cranial cavity) 20
1.4 **Upper jaw, ventro-dorsal**
(oblique projection, open mouth) 22
1.5 **Upper jaw, dorso-ventral**
(superior teeth, nasal cavity) 24
1.6 **Upper jaw, medio-lateral**
(oblique projection, one upper jaw without superimposition) 26
1.7 **Lower jaw, medio-lateral**
(oblique projection, lower jaw without superimposition) 27
1.8 **Bulla tympanica, ventro-dorsal**
(Tympanic bullae, symmetrically) 28

2 Vertebral column (H. WAIBL, E. MAYRHOFER)

2.1 **Cervical vertebral column, latero-lateral**
(extended cervical spine) 30
2.2 **1st and 2nd cervical vertebrae, rostro-caudal,** open mouth
(atlas, axis, dens) 32
2.3 **Cervical vertebral column, ventro-dorsal**
(symmetric vertebral column) 34

General remarks on myelography (E. MAYRHOFER) 37

2.4 **Myelography, Thoracic and lumbar vertebral column,
latero-lateral** 38
2.5 **Myelography, Thoracic and lumbar vertebral column,
ventro-dorsal** 40

3 Thoracic limb (H. WAIBL, L. BRUNNBERG)

3.1 **Shoulder joint, medio-lateral**
(shoulder joint without superimposition) 42
3.2 **Shoulder joint, caudo-cranial**
(articular surfaces) 43
3.3 **Arm, medio-lateral**
(including shoulder and elbow joints) 44
3.4 **Arm, caudo-cranial**
(including shoulder and elbow joints) 45
3.5 **Elbow joint, medio-lateral**
(humeral condyle, olecranon, radial head,
medial coronoid process) 46
3.6 **Elbow joint, cranio-caudal**
(horizontal joint space, humeral condyle) 47
3.7 **Forearm, medio-lateral**
(including elbow and carpal joints) 48
3.8 **Forearm, cranio-caudal**
(including elbow and carpal joints) 49
3.9 **Forepaw, medio-lateral**
(carpal joint, metacarpal bones and digiti, lateral) 50
3.10 **Forepaw, dorso-palmar**
(carpal joint, metacarpal bones and digiti) 51

Postnatal development

Table 3.1 53

3.11 **Shoulder joint, medio-lateral**
(epi- and apophyses) 54
3.12 **Shoulder joint, caudo-cranial**
(epi- and apophyses) 54
3.13 **Elbow joint, medio-lateral**
(epi- and apophyses) 55
3.14 **Elbow joint, cranio-caudal**
(epi- and apophyses) 55
3.15 **Carpal joint, medio-lateral**
(epiphyses) 56
3.16 **Forepaw, dorso-palmar**
(epiphyses, sesamoid bones) 56

4 Pelvic limb (H. WAIBL, U. MATIS, R. KÖSTLIN)

4.1 **Pelvis, latero-lateral**
(survey radiograph) 58
4.2 **Pelvis, latero-lateral**
(oblique projection, pelvic joint without superimposition) 60
4.3 **Pelvis, ventro-dorsal**
(symmetric survey radiograph) 62
4.4 **Pelvis, ventro-dorsal**
(radiograph of one sacroiliac joint) 64
4.5 **Thigh, medio-lateral**
(including hip and stifle joints) 66
4.6 **Thigh, cranio-caudal**
(including hip and stifle joints) 67
4.7 **Stifle joint, medio-lateral**
(including sesamoid bones) 68
4.8 **Stifle joint, cranio-caudal**
(including sesamoid bones) 69
4.9 **Lower leg, medio-lateral**
(including stifle joint and proximal part of the hock joint) 70
4.10 **Lower leg, cranio-caudal**
(including stifle joint and proximal part of the hock joint) 71
4.11 **Hindpaw, medio-lateral**
(survey radiograph, adjacent structures of tibia and fibula) 72
4.12 **Hindpaw, dorso-plantar**
(survey radiograph, adjacent structures of tibia and fibula) 74

Postnatal Development

Table 4.1 77

4.13 **Pelvis and hip joint, ventro-dorsal**
(hip bone, epi- and apophyses) 78
4.14 **Stifle joint, medio-lateral**
(epi- and apophyses, sesamoid bones) 79
4.15 **Stifle joint, cranio-caudal**
(epi- and apophyses, sesamoid bones) 79
4.16 **Hock joint, medio-lateral**
(epi- and apophyses) 80
4.17 **Hindpaw, dorso-plantar**
(epi- and apophyses, sesamoid bones) 80

5 Thorax (H. WAIBL, E. MAYRHOFER)

5.1 **Thorax, latero-lateral**
(thoracic organs) 82
5.2 **Thorax, ventro-dorsal**
(thoracic organs) 84
5.3 **Angiocardiography, latero-lateral**
(endphase of systole, venous side) 86
5.4 **Angiocardiography, latero-lateral**
(diastole, arterial side) 88

6 Abdomen (H. WAIBL, E. MAYRHOFER)

- 6.1 **Abdomen, latero-lateral**
  (survey radiograph) 90
- 6.2 **Abdomen, ventro-dorsal**
  (survey radiograph) 92

Esophageal, gastric and intestinal contrast study
(E. MAYRHOFER) 95

- 6.3 **Contrast, Stomach, Intestine, latero-lateral**
  (gastric wall, duodenum) 96
- 6.4 **Contrast, Stomach, Intestine, ventro-dorsal**
  (gastric wall, pylorus, duodenum) 98
- 6.5 **Contrast, Intestine, latero-lateral**
  (stomach, parts of intestine) 100
- 6.6 **Contrast, Intestine, ventro-dorsal**
  (radiographic study, intestine) 102

- 6.7 **Cholecystography, gallbladder, latero-lateral**
  (radiographic study) 104
- 6.8 **Cholecystography, gallbladder, ventro-dorsal**
  (radiographic study) 106

General remarks on excretory urography (Pyelocystography)
(E. MAYRHOFER) 109

- 6.9 **Pyelography, latero-lateral**
  (renal pelvis, ureter) 110
- 6.10 **Pyelography, ventro-dorsal**
  (renal pelvis, ureter) 112
- 6.11 **Cystography, latero-lateral**
  (negative- and positive-contrast, urinary bladder) 114

7 References 117

Vorwort zur 1. Neuauflage

Nach dem Ableben unseres verehrten Lehrers Prof. Dr. Dr. h. c. Horst Schebitz (München) und der Emeritierung unseres geschätzten, väterlichen Freundes und Ratgebers Prof. Dr. Helmut Wilkens (Hannover) war der außerordentlich erfolgreiche „Schebitz/Wilkens: Atlas der Röntgenanatomie von Hund und Katze" nach einigen Jahren vergriffen. Die besondere Beliebtheit dieses „Kochbuches des Röntgenlabors" im deutschsprachigen Raum und – weil zweisprachig – auch im angloamerikanischen Bereich erforderte eine Neuauflage.

Es sollte jedoch das Buch getrennt für die beiden Tierarten aufgelegt werden; im Jahre 2003 der „Atlas der Röntgenanatomie des Hundes". 2004 wird nun der „Atlas der Röntgenanatomie der Katze" fertig.

Prof. Dr. Wilkens übergab die Herausgeberrechte an mich, seinen Nachfolger am Anatomischen Institut der Tierärztlichen Hochschule in Hannover. Dieser bat im Einvernehmen mit dem Verlag erfahrene befreundete Kollegen aus dem klinischen Bereich um Mitwirkung bei der Neuerstellung des Werkes.

So wurden für einzelne Kapitel die Radiologin Frau Prof. Dr. Elisabeth Mayrhofer (Wien) sowie die Kliniker Frau Prof. Dr. Ulrike Matis und Herr Prof. Dr. Roberto Köstlin (beide München) sowie Herr Prof. Dr. Leo Brunnberg (Berlin) gewonnen.

Wir verdanken die technische Bearbeitung der farbigen Röntgenskizzen und Legenden der gewissenhaften Akribie von Frau Ines Blume, Frau Gudrun Wirth und Frau Marlis Bewarder (Hannover) sowie die erfolgreiche Umarbeitung der Lagerungsskizzen dem Können der akademischen Zeichnerin Frau Caren-Imme von Stemm (Hannover). Frau Dr. Sibylle Kneissl (Wien) übernahm die englische Übersetzung, die von Prof. Dr. James E. Smallwood (Raleigh, North Carolina) dankenswerterweise durchgesehen wurde.

Dem Parey Verlag Stuttgart sei hier ausdrücklich für die hervorragende Förderung und die gute Zusammenarbeit bei der Herstellung dieses Werkes gedankt. Stellvertretend sei hier namentlich Frau Dr. Ines George genannt.

Das Buch ist eine „Röntgenanatomie der Katze", die dem praktizierenden Kollegium bei der Beurteilung der selbst angefertigten Röntgenbilder eine Grundlage zur Interpretation bilden soll.

Hannover, im Winter 2003/2004   Helmut Waibl

Preface to the 1st new edition

A few years after the death of our much-admired teacher Prof. Dr. Dr. h. c. Horst Schebitz (Munich) and the retirement of our esteemed, fatherly friend and advisor Prof. Dr. Helmut Wilkens (Hanover), the very successful "Schebitz/Wilkens: Atlas of Radiographic Anatomy of the Dog and Cat" went out of print. The special popularity of this "cook-book of the radiological laboratory" in the German- and English-speaking countries made a new edition necessary.

However, the new book was to be published separately for each species; first, in 2003, the "Atlas of Radiographic Anatomy of the Dog", and then, in 2004, the "Atlas of Radiographic Anatomy of the Cat" will be finished.

Prof. Dr. Wilkens handed over the editor's rights to me, his succeeder at the Institute of Anatomy of the School of Veterinary Medicine Hanover. In agreement with the publisher, I asked experienced colleagues working in the clinical field to cooperate. Therefore the radiologist Prof. Dr. Elisabeth Mayrhofer (Vienna) and the clinicians Prof. Dr. Ulrike Matis (Munich), Prof. Dr. Roberto Köstlin (Munich) and Prof. Dr. Leo Brunnberg (Berlin) agreed to contribute chapters to this new edition.

Many thanks go to Ines Blume, Gudrun Wirth, Marlis Bewarder (Hanover) and Caren-Imme von Stemm (Hanover). Mrs. Wirth, Mrs. Blume and Mrs. Bewarder processed the x-ray sketches and legends in a very precise way and Mrs. von Stemm, an academic designer, worked over the positioning sketches very successfully. Further thanks go to Dr. Sibylle Kneissl (Vienna), who translated the new chapters into English, and to Prof. Dr. James E. Smallwood (Raleigh, North Carolina) for his supervision of the translation.

Special recognition must be accorded to Parey Verlag Stuttgart for the excellent promotion and cooperation during the production of this book. Dr. Ines George should be named representatively.

This book is a "radiographic anatomy of the cat", intended to provide the practitioner with basic information for interpreting x-ray images.

Hanover, winter 2003/2004   Helmut Waibl

Einführung

Der vorliegende Atlas hat sich, verglichen mit den entsprechenden Abschnitten seines Vorläufers **(Schebitz/Wilkens: Atlas der Röntgenanatomie von Hund und Katze, 5. Auflage, 1989)**, doch deutlich verändert.
Was ist neu ?

a) Inhalt

Dieser Atlas ist nur noch der **Röntgenanatomie der Katze** zur gezielten Anwendung in der Praxis gewidmet.
Neue Röntgendarstellungen (1.8, 2.4, 2.5) wurden eingefügt.

b) Lagerungen

Allgemeines zu Lagerungen ist einführend (S. 12) zusammengefasst. Insbesondere wird die Fixierung der Katzen – in Abhängigkeit von den jeweils gültigen Röntgenschutzverordnungen – nur beispielhaft dargestellt und ihre Anwendung bei der Röntgenaufnahme der Verantwortung des behandelnden Tierarztes überlassen.

Die Lagerungsskizzen (mit Kassette sowie dem Kegel der Nutzstrahlen) werden jeder einzelnen Röntgendarstellung direkt zugeordnet. Damit wird das Suchen und Blättern im Buch vermieden.

Diesen Lagerungsskizzen sind hilfreiche Anmerkungen und Beachtungshinweise direkt beigegeben.

c) Röntgenskizzen

Hier wurden die wichtigen Details (Einzelknochen oder Organe) mit unterschiedlichen Farben dargestellt, um eine schnellere Orientierung zu gewinnen. Dabei kennzeichnet dieselbe Farbe – wo dies möglich ist – dunkel die plattennahen Strukturen und heller die plattenfernen Strukturen. Manchmal musste dies durch die Legendenbezeichnung (z.B. A und A' = plattenfern) gekennzeichnet werden.

Wichtiger war bei der Bearbeitung der Skizzen die Verringerung der Buchstaben und Ziffern in den Skizzen (und damit auch in den Legenden) um etwa die Hälfte ohne Informationsverlust! Dieses "Ausmerzen von Beschriftungen" in den Skizzen wurde – insbesondere an der Wirbelsäule – weitergeführt, da hier z.B. nur bestimmte Wirbel hervorgehoben wurden. Zudem wurden die Buchstaben farblich den Legendenteilen zugeordnet. Damit hoffen wir den Wunsch aus der Kollegenschaft nach Übersichtlichkeit erfüllt zu haben.

Die Röntgenskizzen zur postnatalen Entwicklung der Extremitätenknochen wurden modifiziert und dabei die Epi- und Apophysen sowie die Sesambeine farblich differenziert. Diese Maßnahme sollte gerade bei der Interpretation der Röntgenbilder von Katzen im 1. (und 2.) Lebensjahr hilfreich sein.

d) Legenden der Röntgenskizzen

Die anatomischen Fachausdrücke in den Legenden entsprechen farblich der Nummerierung in den Skizzen. Diese Termini technici sind der international gültigen Nomina Anatomica Veterinaria (NAV 1994) entnommen.

Introduction

This atlas is distinctly different from its precursor **(Schebitz/Wilkens: Atlas of Radiographic Anatomy of the Dog and Cat, 5th edition, 1989).**
What is new?

a) Content

This atlas is only dedicated to the practical use of **radiographic anatomy of the cat**.
New x-ray images (1.8, 2.4, 2.5) were inserted.

b) Positioning

General remarks on positioning techniques were summarized at the beginning of this book (p. 13). Different methods of fixation – legally regulated – are illustrated; the method applied is left to the competence of the treating veterinarian.

For a better orientation positioning sketches are attached to each x-ray image.

Further helpful remarks and suggestions are added to the sketches.

c) X-ray sketches

Relevant details (bones or organs) are illustrated in different colors in order to provide a better reference. Dark colors mark structures near the plate, bright colors mark structures near the tube. Sometimes this had to be included in the legend (i.e. A and A' = next to the tube).

To get a better overview, letters and numbers on x-ray sketches were reduced by half. To achieve this without loss of information, fewer structures, i.e. certain vertebrae, were marked and a colored codification was used.

The x-ray sketches of the postnatal development were modified. Epi- and apophyses as well as sesamoids were differentiated using colors. This should greatly assist in the interpretation of x-ray images in the juvenile cat.

d) Legends of the x-ray sketches

The colored numbers of the anatomical terms in the legends correspond to the color used in the sketches. The nomenclature used in this atlas is based on the Nomina Anatomica Veterinaria (NAV 1994).

Allgemeines zur Lagerung

Die Röntgenverordnungen in den verschiedenen Ländern bedingen hohe Sicherheitsstufen für das Personal, evtl. begleitende Tierbesitzer und die Patienten im Röntgenraum. Folglich existieren einige grundsätzliche Sicherheitsregeln:

> Der durchstrahlte Bereich ist so klein wie möglich, aber so groß wie nötig zu wählen.
> In bestimmten Ländern werden alle Katzen in Vollnarkose geröntgt.
> Da sich Katzen ungern einem Zwang fügen, der für eine korrekte Lagerung jedoch notwendig sein kann, sind Röntgenaufnahmen mit Geduld und Einfühlungsvermögen oder mit einer rechtzeitig vorgenommenen Sedierung durchzuführen.
> Grundsätzlich dürfen **fixierende Hände nicht im Kegel der Nutzstrahlen** sein.
> Wenn ein Tier gehalten werden muss (unter Beachtung der gültigen Strahlenschutzverordnungen), sind unbedingt Bleigummihandschuhe zu tragen.
> Diese und weitere Schutzbekleidung schützen lediglich vor der energieärmeren Streustrahlung!
> Somit sind eventuelle Haltepunkte möglichst weit entfernt vom Nutzstrahlenbündel zu wählen.

Um diesen Sicherheitsbestimmungen zu entsprechen, sind im Folgenden 3 Beispiele einer Röntgenaufnahme des Abdomens in der rechten Seitenlagerung einer Katze ohne und mit Fixierungen demonstriert.

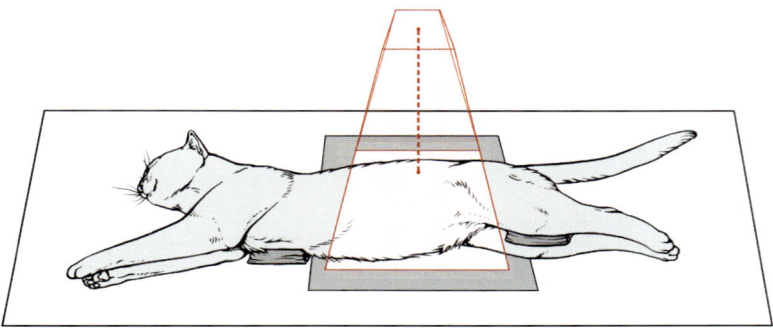

Abb. 1a Rechte Seitenlage einer Katze ohne Fixierung.
Schaumstoffkeile unter dem Sternum und zwischen den Kniegelenken gewähren eine exakte Lagerung ohne Rotationen. (Die notwendige Streckung des Patienten ist so kaum zu erreichen.)

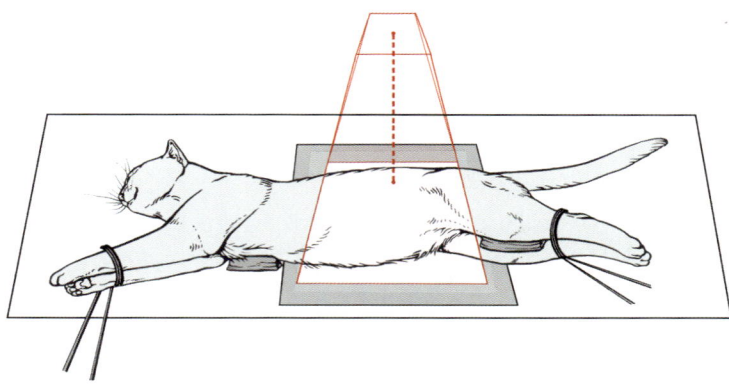

Abb. 1c Rechte Seitenlagerung einer Katze mit Fixierung durch Bänder an den Extremitäten.
Unter den Thorax und zwischen die Kniegelenke sind Schaumstoffkeile gelegt.

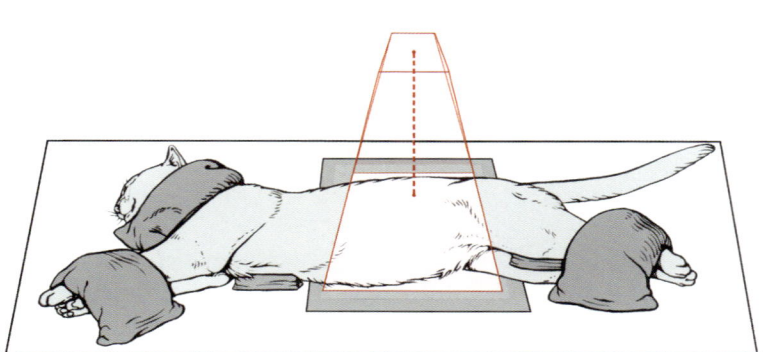

Abb. 1b Rechte Seitenlagerung einer Katze mit Fixierung durch Sandsäcke am Hals und an den Extremitäten.
Unter den Thorax und zwischen die Kniegelenke sind Schaumstoffkeile gelegt.

Selbstverständlich existieren viele unterschiedliche Lagerungs- und Fixierungsmöglichkeiten der Patienten. Hierzu finden Sie bei jedem Röntgenbild eine Lagerungsskizze mit beachtenswerten Hilfen.

Die für den Patienten notwendige Fixierungsart muss – aus den oben genannten Gründen – dem behandelnden Tierarzt überlassen bleiben, da nur er den Zustand bzw. die Belastbarkeit des Patienten beurteilen kann und letztlich für die korrekte Röntgenuntersuchung unter den gesetzlichen Vorschriften verantwortlich ist!

General remarks on positioning

Radiation safety regulations were designed to protect both radiation workers and patients. In the following you will find basic radiation safety rules for diagnostic radioglogy:

> The exposure area should be no larger than is necessary to include the region of interest.
>
> In some countries radiological examinations are performed under general anesthesia.
>
> Because cats do not like being held in one position for very long, positioning of cats for radiography requires either a good deal of patience or some level of sedation.
>
> Always wear protective gloves, when holding an animal and observe the valid radiation safety regulations.
>
> **Never permit fixing hands, even if gloved, to be in the primary beam.**
>
> Lead-lined gloves and additional protective clothing are designed to protect only against low-energy, scattered radiation!
>
> Choose fixation points as far as possible from the primary beam.

In the following, 3 examples of an x-ray image in right lateral recumbency with and without fixation are given and demonstrate the above rules.

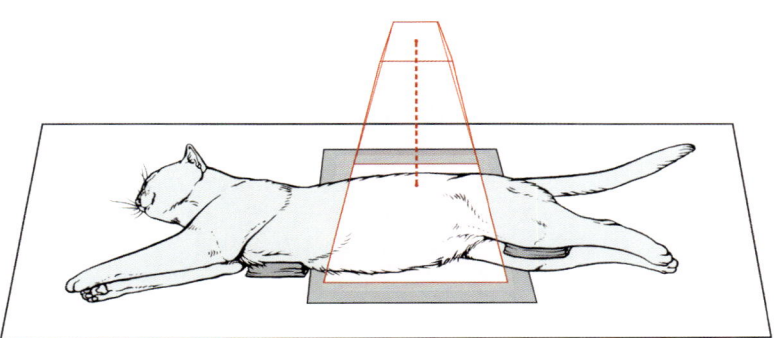

Fig. 1a   Right lateral recumbency of a cat without fixation.
Foam wedges supporting the sternum and nondependent stifle allow an accurate positioning without rotation. (Full extension of the patient cannot be achieved.)

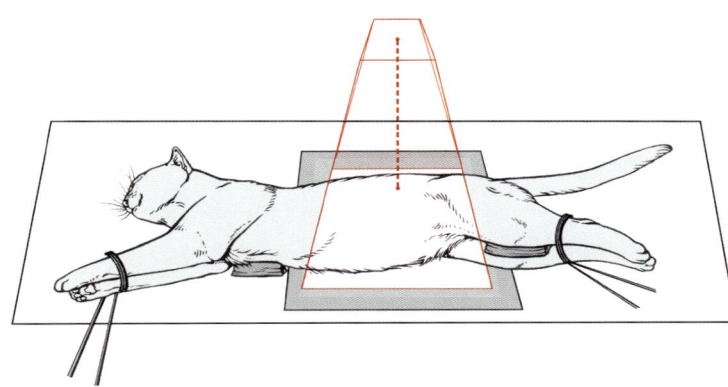

Fig. 1c   Right lateral recumbency of a cat with fixation. Ribbons were attached to the extremities.
Foam wedges support thorax and the nondependent stifle.

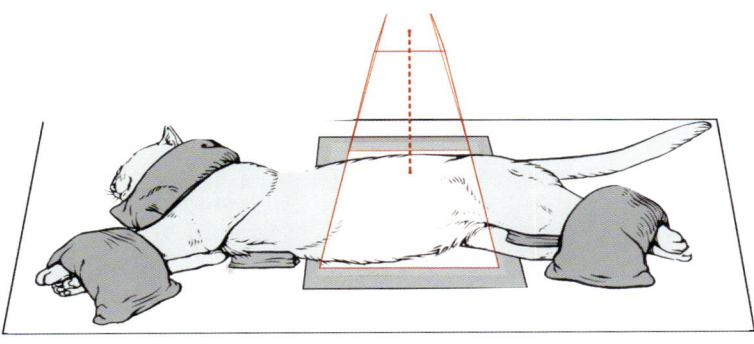

Fig. 1b   Right lateral recumbency of a cat with fixation. Sandbags were placed on neck and distal extremities.
Foam wedges support thorax and the nondependent stifle.

Naturally, there are many different methods of positioning and fixation. Therefore you will find helpful positioning sketches for each x-ray image.

The method of choice is left to the competence of the attending veterinarian, as the veterinarian, not the assistant, is the person responsible for adherence to the radiation safety regulations as well as for the condition and behavior of the patient.

Hinweise für die Belichtung von Röntgenaufnahmen

Viele Faktoren beeinflussen die Entstehung eines Röntgenbildes; daher ist es nicht möglich, eine allgemein gültige „Belichtungstabelle" zu erstellen. Die Kenntnis der Faktoren und generelle Richtlinien erlauben jedoch, relativ schnell eine individuelle Tabelle zu erhalten. Die Vorschrift des Strahlenschutzgesetzes, dass die Belichtungsdaten jedes Bildes notiert werden müssen, erleichtert diese Maßnahme.

Einfluss auf die **Bildschwärzung** nehmen neben den gewählten kV und mAs der Fokus-Film-Abstand (FFA), die Objektdicke und -beschaffenheit, das Film-Folienmaterial, die Verwendung von Rastern und die Qualität der Entwicklung.

Die gewählte **Spannung (kV)** beeinflusst die Wellenlänge und damit die Durchdringungsfähigkeit der Röntgenstrahlen. Die üblichen Röntgenapparate bieten 50–100 kV an. 50 kV sind relativ energiearm und wenig durchdringungsfähig. Sie werden vom Objekt relativ leicht absorbiert und verursachen dann keine Schwärzung des Röntgenfilmes. Das bedeutet, dass sie nur bei dünnen bzw. strahlendurchlässigen Objekten verwendet werden sollten. Eine Spannung von 100 kV hingegen bedeutet energiereiche, hoch durchdringungsfähige Röntgenstrahlung. Teile der Strahlung werden jedoch absorbiert, die Reststrahlung breitet sich mit verminderter Energie in alle Richtungen des Raumes aus. Diese Sekundär- oder Streustrahlung belastet die Umgebung (Strahlenschutz!) und verschlechtert die Bildqualität durch Schrägprojektionen, das Bild wird „grau" und weniger scharf. Für Katzen werden im Allgemeinen 50–65 V ausreichend sein, d.h., die Streustrahlung ist relativ gering, und es kann ohne Raster gearbeitet werden.

Die **Milliampere (mA)** geben die Stromstärke und damit die Leistungsfähigkeit des Röntgenapparates an. Je höher der Heizstrom für die Glühkathode, umso mehr Elektronen und letztlich Bremsstrahlen stehen zur Verfügung. Da immer nur das **mAs-Produkt** wirksam wird, können viel mA mit wenig s denselben Wert ergeben wie wenig mA x viel s. Bei längerer Belichtungszeit ist jedoch mit Bewegungsunschärfen zu rechnen.

kV und **mAs** stehen in gewisser Abhängigkeit zueinander: Man erzielt eine vergleichbare Bildschwärzung bei Erhöhung der kV und Reduktion der mAs. Als Richtwert gilt:

> plus 10 kV verlangen die halben mAs-Werte,
> minus 10 kV das doppelte mAs-Produkt.

Der **Fokus-Film-Abstand** beträgt im Allgemeinen 70–100 cm. Entsprechend dem „Abstandquadratgesetz" verringert sich die Intensität der Röntgenstrahlen mit dem Quadrat der Entfernungszunahme.

Nicht nur die **Dicke des Objektes**, sondern auch seine Zusammensetzung muss berücksichtigt werden: Lungengewebe schwächt die Röntgenstrahlen weniger als Parenchyme, Muskeln oder gar Knochen.

Je dicker und dichter das Objekt, umso höhere kV müssen gewählt werden; dies erhöht die Streustrahlung und damit die Strahlenbelastung der Umgebung. Die Bildqualität verschlechtert sich.

Ab einer Objektdicke von etwa 15 cm ist die Verwendung eines **Rasters** empfehlenswert; es wird zwischen Objekt und Röntgenkassette eingebracht. Die darin enthaltenen Bleilamellen absorbieren ungerichtete Strahlung, aber auch einen Teil der Primärstrahlung, weshalb die mAs um den Rasterfaktor, meist 2–3, erhöht werden müssen. Die Bildqualität wird wesentlich verbessert, doch die Aufnahmezeit verlängert. Die Röntgenstrahlen müssen exakt senkrecht auf das Raster fallen, und die am Raster angegebene Distanz zum Fokus muss eingehalten werden. Praktisch bedeutet das, ein Raster kann höchstens bei extrem dicken Katzen sinnvoll sein.

In den **Röntgenkassetten** befinden sich zwei Verstärkerfolien, die Röntgenstrahlen in Licht des blauen oder grünen Spektralbereiches umwandeln. Der beidseitig beschichtete **Film** wird durch dieses Licht und die restliche Röntgenstrahlung geschwärzt. Wichtig ist, dass Filme und Verstärkerfolien zusammenpassen. Die gemeinsame Wirkung wird in „Empfindlichkeitsklassen" definiert, dadurch werden die unterschiedlichsten Kombinationen vergleichbar. Die Empfindlichkeitsklasse 200 benötigt z. B. die doppelte Dosis der Klasse 400.

Verstärkerfolien werden als
- **feinzeichnend** = bei dünnen Objekten, mit guter Detailerkennbarkeit und relativ viel Dosis,
- **hochverstärkend** = bei dicken Objekten, mit schlechterer Detailerkennbarkeit und relativ geringer Dosis oder als
- **Standard-** bzw. **Universalfolie** als Kompromiss aus den vorgenannten Folien angeboten.
- **Seltene Erden-Folien** sparen bei dicken Objekten Dosis und erreichen eine gute Auflösung. Für Katzen ist im Allgemeinen ein 200er bis maximal 400er System ausreichend, bei geringen kV-Werten sind relativ hohe mA-Werte gegeben, die Belichtungszeit kann daher sehr kurz gewählt werden. Feinzeichnende und Standard-Folien sind für viele Röntgenaufnahmen der Katze ausreichend.

Der **Entwicklungsvorgang** muss exakt und genormt sein. Temperatur, Zeit der Entwicklung und Alter der Entwicklerlösung haben einen großen Einfluss auf die Bildschwärzung.

Wenn man sich bemüht, möglichst viele Faktoren konstant zu halten (FFA, Film-Folienqualität, Entwicklung), muss man die kV und mAs nur noch dem Objekt anpassen.

Am **Tierkörper** selbst gibt es vergleichbare **Regionen**, welche die Belichtung ebenfalls vereinfachen. So brauchen i. A.
- Wirbelsäule, Abdomen und Becken die gleichen Werte,
- Kopf, Hals, Thorax etwas weniger.

Folgende Regionen sind in den Röntgendosiswerten gleichzusetzen:
- Oberarm und Oberschenkel,
- Ellbogen- und Kniegelenke,
- Unterarm und Unterschenkel sowie
- Karpus, Tarsus und Phalangen.

Belichtungstabelle für Röntgenaufnahmen bei der Katze
FFD = 75 cm; Empfindlichkeitsklasse: 400; maschinelle Entwicklung (30 °C)

Region	kV/mAs	Region	kV/mAs
Kopf LL	55/1,25	Schultergelenk KK	55/1,25
Kopf DV	55/1,25	Oberarm LL	55/1,25
HWS LL	55/1,25	Oberarm KK	55/1,25
HWS VD	55/1,25	Ellbogengelenk LL	52/1,25
BWS LL	58/1,25	Ellbogengelenk KK	52/1,25
BWS VD	58/1,25	Unterarm LL	52/1,25
LWS LL	58/1,25	Unterarm KK	52/1,25
LWS VD	62/1,25	Handwurzel - Pfote	50/1,25
Becken LL	62/1,25	Oberschenkel LL	55/1,25
Becken VD	65/1,25	Oberschenkel KK	58/1,25
Thorax LL	55/1,25	Kniegelenk LL	52/1,25
Thorax DV	58/1,25	Kniegelenk KK	52/1,25
Abdomen LL	62/1,25	Unterschenkel LL	52/1,25
Abdomen VD	65/1,25	Unterschenkel KK	52/1,25
Schultergelenk LL	55/1,25	Fußwurzel – Pfote	50/1,25

FFD = Fokus-Film-Distanz KK = kaudo-kranial DV = dorso-ventral
LL = latero-lateral kranio-kaudal VD = ventro-dorsal.

Comments on the exposure of x-ray images

Because many factors influence the formation of an x-ray image, it is not possible to provide generally accurate exposure data. However, knowledge of those factors and general guidelines allow us to gain an individual set of exposure data in a relatively short time. This is supported by a law that requires the documentation of exposure data for every x-ray procedure performed.

Film opacity is influenced by x-ray tube kilovoltage and milliamperage, focal-film distance (FFD), thickness, composition of the tissue, film and screen characteristics, applied grids, and the quality of film processing.

The applied **voltage (kV)** influences the wavelength of the x-rays and thus their penetration power. Conventional x-ray units offer 50–100 kV. An x-ray beam of 50 kV has relatively low energy and therefore little penetrating power. The x-rays will likely be absorbed by the object and thus produce no film density. This means, that low voltage should be applied to image thin, radiation-transmitting objects only. However, high voltage of 100 kV produces high-energy radiation of high penetration power. Parts of the radiation are attenuated, the remaining radiation propagates with less energy in all directions. This secondary or scattered radiation affects the environment (mind radiation safety!) and decreases image quality due to oblique projections. The image is "gray" and less sharp. In general, 50–65 kV are adequate to penetrate the body of the cat, which means secondary radiation is relatively low and the use of a grid is not necessary.

X-ray tube current, measured in **milliamperes (mA)**, refers to the capacity of the x-ray tube. The higher the tube current for the filament, the more electrons are available, and the more x-rays produced. Because the **mAs product** is what is really important, high mA and a short time is equal to a longer time and less mA. The major disadvantage is that longer exposure times increase the likelihood of motion artifact during the exposure.

kV and mAs are dependent on each other: Similar film density is achieved by increasing kV and reducing mAs. There reference value is:

> A 10 kV increase requires half of the mAs value, or a 10 kV reduction requires doubling of the mAs.

Focal-film distance varies from 70 to 100 cm; according to the inverse square law the intensity of the x-ray beam per unit area is inversely related to the square of the distance from the focal spot of the x-ray tube.

Attenuation of the x-ray beam traversing an **object** depends on the thickness of the object as well as its tissue composition: lung tissue attenuates x-rays less than parenchyma, muscle or bone of the same thickness.

KV must be increased with greater thickness and density of the object; this leads to more scattered radiation, which contributes to more exposure of the patient and to more film fog.

A **grid** should be used, if the object thickness exceeds 15 cm; it is placed between the object and the x-ray cassette. A radiographic grid consists of a series of lead foils that are most effective in removing scattered radiation with minimal impact on primary radiation. Consequently, exposure factors must be increased according to the grid or Bucky factor, usually 2–3 times the mAs applied without a grid. When using a grid, the focal-film distance must be selected as indicated, and the x-ray beam must be directed perpendicular to the cassette. In summary, a grid increases image contrast, but leads to higher patient exposure. In practice, grids are not necessary when radiographing cats, unless the cat is greater than 15 cm thick.

The x-ray film is sandwiched between two intensifying screens in a **cassette**; these screens convert x-rays into light, primarily in the blue and green wavelengths of the visible spectrum. This light and the x-ray beam produce blackening of the **x-ray film**. It is important, that the film and screen used are matched. The combined effect is defined by "speed classes" in order to make different combinations comparable. Speed class 200, for example, requires double the x-ray dose as does speed class 400.

Intensifying screens are classified by fast, medium and slow. Fast intensifying screens are used to image thick objects. They require less x-ray exposure, but yield decreased image detail. Slow intensifying screens are used to image thin objects. They allow good image detail, but require more x-ray exposure. Medium-speed intensifying screens (standard or universal) are a compromise of the properties mentioned above. New technology has resulted in very fast rare-earth screens, which require less x-ray exposure and provide acceptable image detail. In general, speed class 200 to 400 are recommended for cats, a low kV requires a high mA value, so that exposure time can be reduced. In practice, slow and medium intensifying screens will be adequate for cats.

Film processing needs to be done properly and with a standardized technique. Temperature and developing time, as well as the age of the developing agents, affect film blackening.

If you keep a number of variables (FFD, film and screen quality, film processing) constant, only kV and mAs need to be adjusted to the object.

According to x-ray dose **comparable regions on the animal's body** exist and allow a simplification of the exposure factors. Thus, abdomen and pelvis require the same x-ray dose, while head, neck and thorax need slightly less.

The following regions are comparable according to the x-ray dose:
- Upper arm and thigh,
- elbow and stifle joint,
- forearm and lower leg as well as
- carpus, tarsus and digits.

Exposure data for the radiological examination of the cat
FFD = 75 cm; speed class: 400; automatic film processing (30 °C)

Region	kV / mAs	Region	kV / mAs
head LL	55/1,25	shoulder joint CC	55/1,25
head DV	55/1,25	arm LL	55/1,25
cervical spine LL	55/1,25	arm CC	55/1,25
cervical spine VD	55/1,25	elbow joint LL	52/1,25
thoracic spine LL	58/1,25	elbow joint CC	52/1,25
thoracic spine VD	58/1,25	forearm LL	52/1,25
lumbar spine LL	58/1,25	forearm CC	52/1,25
lumbar spine VD	62/1,25	carpal joint and forepaw	50/1,25
pelvis LL	62/1,25	thigh LL	55/1,25
pelvis VD	65/1,25	thigh CC	58/1,25
thorax LL	55/1,25	stifle joint LL	52/1,25
thorax DV	58/1,25	stifle joint CC	52/1,25
abdomen LL	62/1,25	lower leg LL	52/1,25
abdomen VD	65/1,25	lower leg CC	52/1,25
shoulder joint LL	55/1,25	tarsal joint and hindpaw	50/1,25

FFD = focal-film distance
LL = laterolateral
CC = caudocranial / craniocaudal
DV = dorsoventral
VD = ventrodorsal.

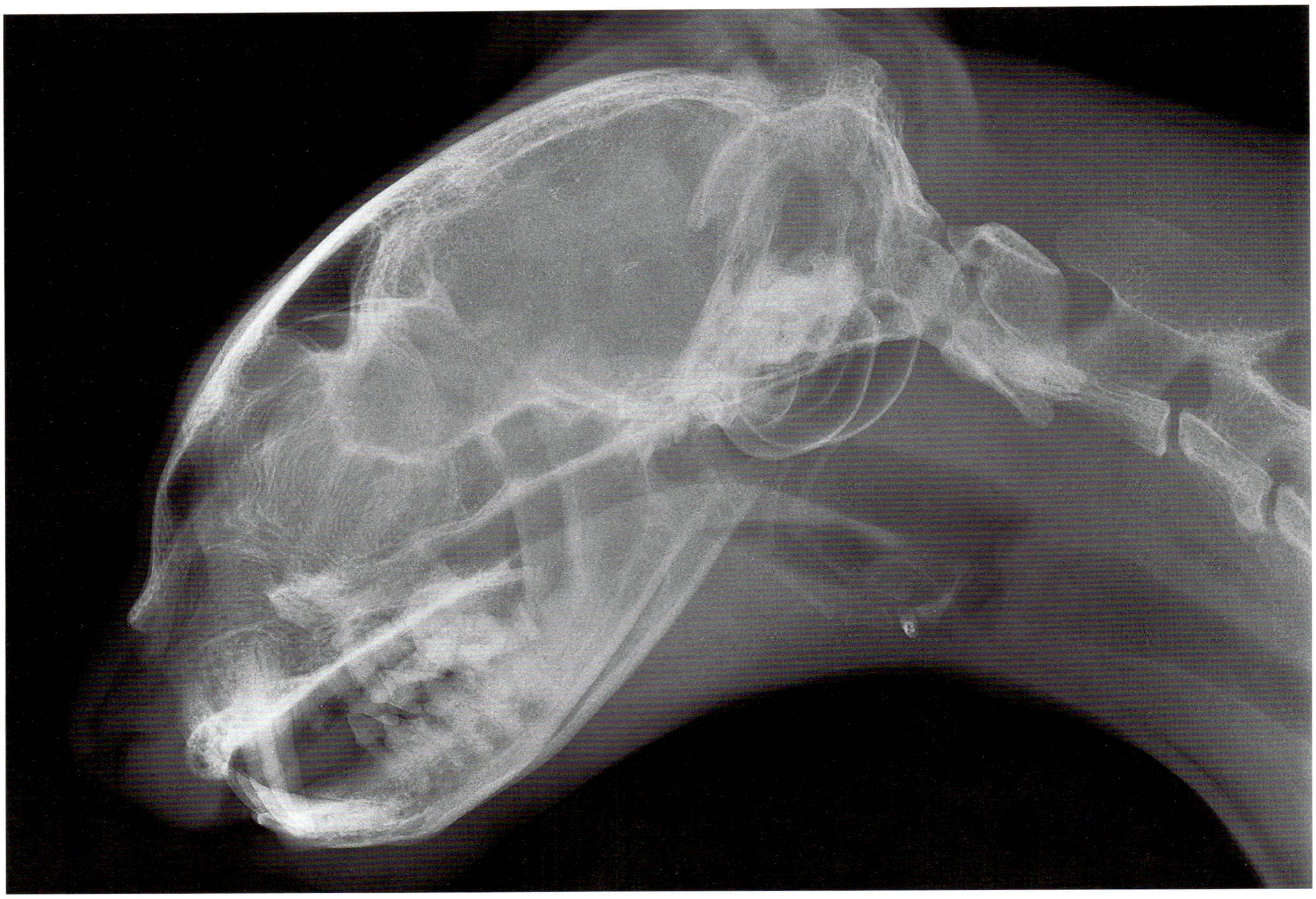

1 Kopf – Head

Abb. 1.1 Kopf, latero-lateral,
Katze
(Ausschnitt aus 13 × 18 cm)

Fig. 1.1 Head, latero-lateral,
Cat
(section of 13 × 18 cm)

■ **Ziel**
Darstellung der Kopfknochen, Schädelhöhle und Bullae tympanicae.

■ **Zentralstrahl**
Senkrecht zur Kassette, in Höhe des Kiefergelenks.

■ **Beachte**
Medianebene des Kopfes parallel zur Kassette. Mit einem Schaumgummikeil unter dem ventro-rostralen Kopfbereich kann der Kopf korrekt gelagert werden.

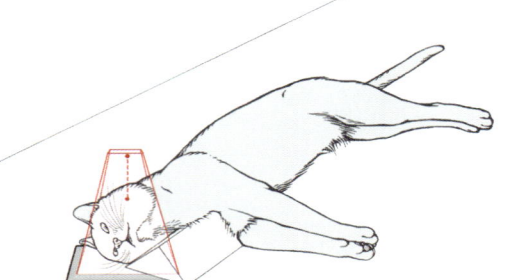

Abb 1.1 Lagerung zur Aufnahme des Kopfes. Latero-lateral.

Fig. 1.1 Positioning of head. Latero-lateral.

■ *Objective*
To obtain a lateral radiographic image of the cranial bones and cranial cavity.

■ *Central ray of the primary beam*
Direct the x-ray beam perpendicular to the cassette, with the central ray centered at the level of the temporo-mandibular joint.

■ *Notice*
Align the median plane of the head parallel to the cassette. Support the rostral part of the head with a foam rubber wedge to position the head correctly.

1.1 Kopf – Head ■ latero-lateral

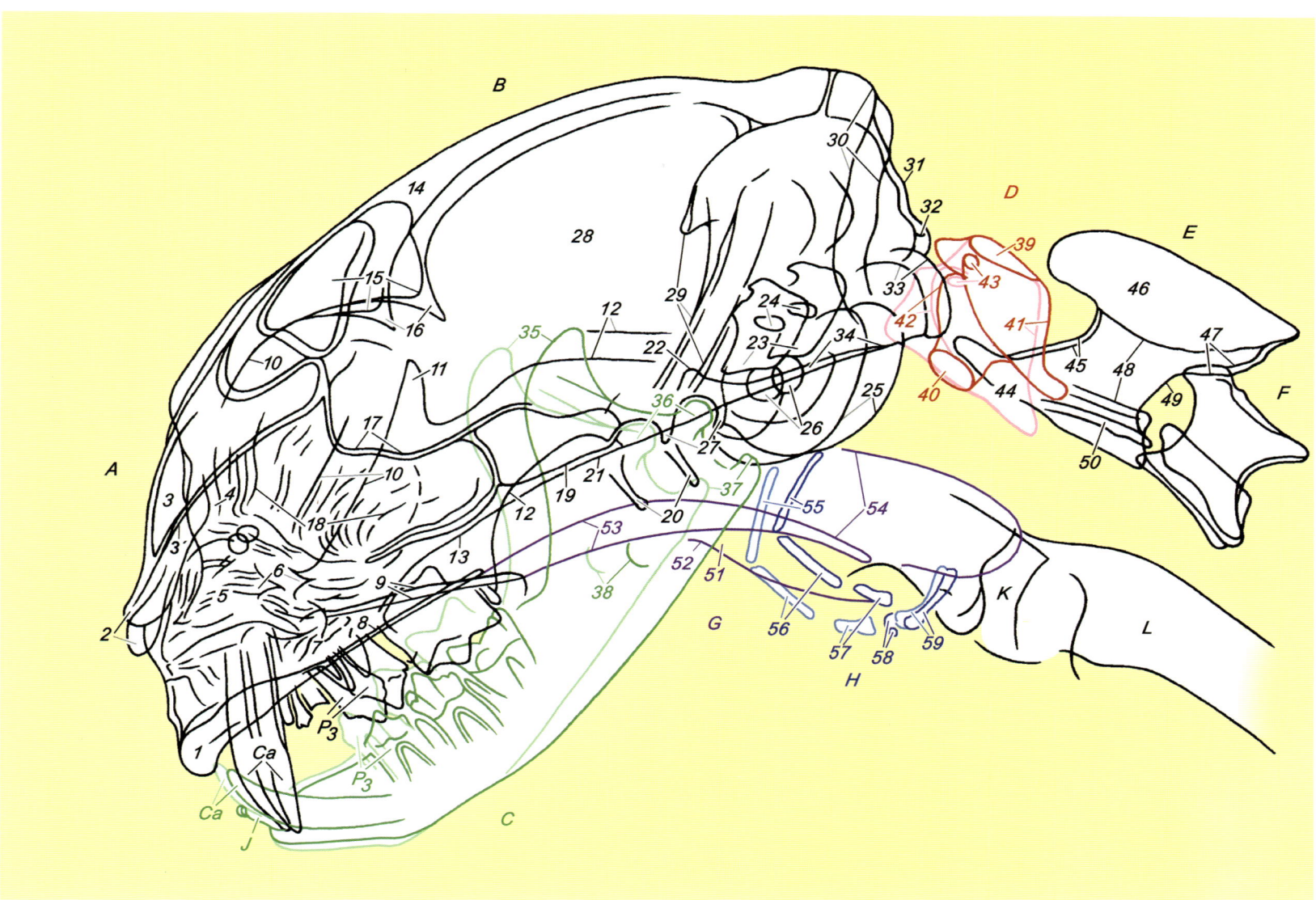

A Ossa faciei
1 Os incisivum
2 Os nasale, Processus rostralis
3 Meatus nasi dorsalis
3´ Crista ethmoidalis
4 Concha nasalis dorsalis
5 Concha nasalis ventralis
6 Foramen infraorbitale
7 Meatus nasi ventralis
8 Palatum durum
9 Orbita, ventrale Begrenzung – *ventral border*
10 Margo infraorbitalis
11 Os zygomaticum, Processus frontalis
12 Arcus zygomaticus, ventraler Rand – *ventral border*
13 Vomer
Ca Dens caninus
P₃ Dens praemolaris III

B Ossa cranii
14 Os frontale
15 Sinus frontalis
16 Os frontale, Processus zygomaticus
17 Fossa ethmoidalis
18 Labyrinthus ethmoidalis
19 Sinus sphenoidalis, ventrale Begrenzung – *ventral border*
20 Hamulus pterygoideus
21 Basis cranii, Os praesphenoidale
22 Dorsum sellae turcicae
23 Os temporale, Pars petrosa
24 Porus acusticus internus
25 Os temporale, Pars tympanica
26 Porus acusticus externus
27 Processus retroarticularis
28 Cavum cranii
29 Tentorium cerebelli osseum
30 Crista nuchae, lateral Crista temporalis
31 Squama occipitalis
32 Foramen magnum, dorsaler Rand – *dorsal border*
33 Condylus occipitalis
34 Os occipitale, Pars basilaris

C Mandibula
35 Processus coronoideus
36 Processus condylaris
37 Processus angularis
38 Foramen mandibulae

Ca Dens caninus

J Dentes incisivi

P₃ Dens praemolaris III

D Atlas
39 Arcus dorsalis
40 Arcus ventralis
41 Ala atlantis
42 Fovea articularis cranialis
43 Foramen vertebrale laterale

E Axis
44 Dens
45 Incisura vertebralis cranialis
46 Processus spinosus
47 Processus articularis caudalis
48 Canalis vertebrae
49 Incisura vertebralis caudalis
50 Processus transversus

F C III

G Pharynx
51 Pars oralis
52 Radix linguae
53 Velum palatinum
54 Pars nasalis

H Os hyoideum
55 Stylohyoideum
56 Epihyoideum
57 Ceratohyoideum
58 Basihyoideum
59 Thyreohyoideum

K Larynx

L Trachea

1 Kopf – Head

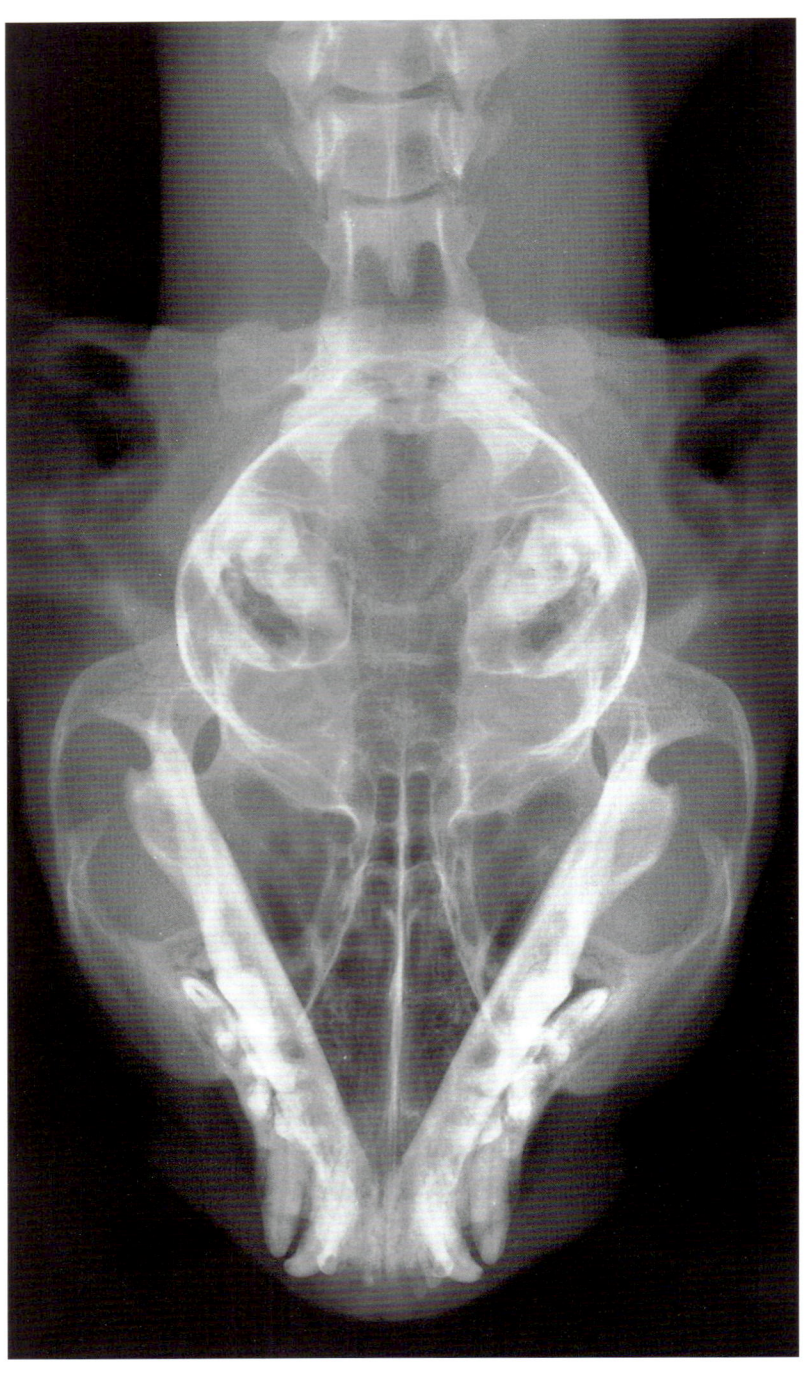

Abb. 1.2 Kopf, ventro-dorsal,
Katze
(Ausschnitt aus 13 × 18 cm)

Fig. 1.2 Head, ventro-dorsal,
Cat
(section of 13 × 18 cm)

■ **Ziel**
Symmetrische Übersichtsaufnahme der Kopfhälften.

■ **Zentralstrahl**
Senkrecht zur Kassette, auf die Medianlinie des Kopfes in Höhe des Angulus mandibulae.

■ **Beachte**
Die Kehlränder des Unterkiefers in gleicher Höhe zur Kassette. Schon eine geringe Verkantung verursacht erhebliche Verzeichnungen und Überlagerungen. Die Lagerung des Nasenrückens lässt sich durch Unterlegen eines Schaumgummikeils unter die ersten Halswirbel erleichtern.

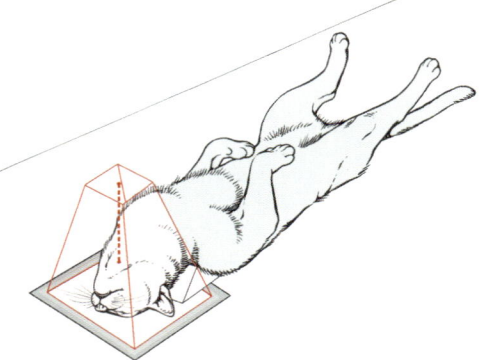

Abb. 1.2 Lagerung zur Aufnahme des Kopfes. Nasenrücken anliegend. Ventro-dorsal.

Fig. 1.2 Positioning of head with dorsum nasi resting on cassette. Ventro-dorsal.

■ *Objective*
To obtain a symmetric ventro-dorsal radiographic image of the head.

■ *Central ray of the primary beam*
Direct the x-ray beam perpendicular to the cassette, with the central ray centered on the median plane at the level of the angle of the mandible.

■ *Notice*
Position the head with the ventral borders of the mandibles at the same level. Even a slight tilting of the head causes considerable distortion and superimposition.
To facilitate positioning, support the more cranial cervical vertebrae with a foam rubber wedge.

1.2 Kopf – Head ■ ventro-dorsal

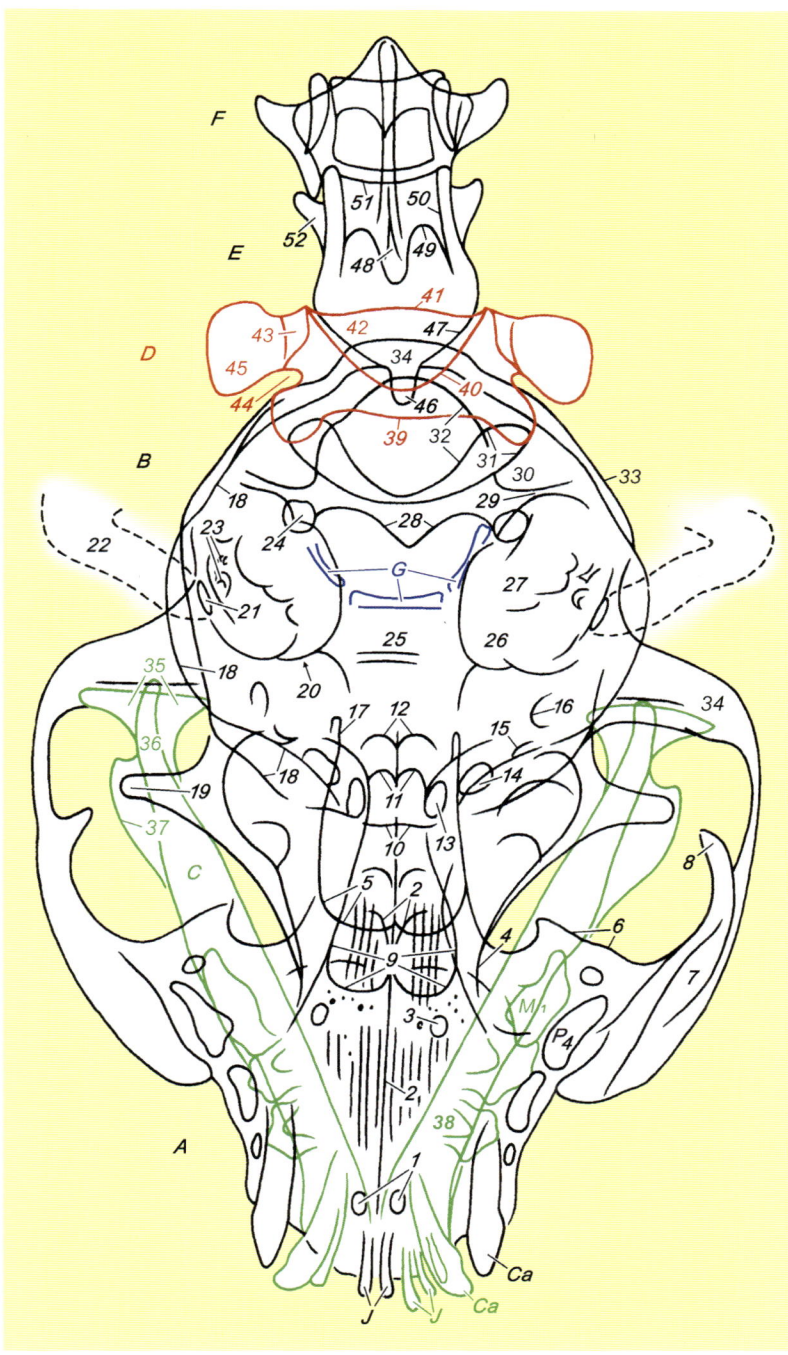

A Ossa faciei
1. Fissura palatina
2. Sutura palatina mediana et Vomer
3. Foramen sphenopalatinum
4. Orbita, mediale Wand – *medial wall*
5. Choanenrand mit Spina nasalis caudalis – *border of Choana with Spina nasalis caudalis*
6. Os maxillare, kaudaler Rand – *caudal border*
7. Os zygomaticum, Processus temporalis
8. Os zygomaticum, Processus frontalis

J Dentes incisivi
Ca Dens caninus
P₄ Dens praemolaris IV

B Ossa cranii
9. Fossa ethmoidalis
10. Crista orbitosphenoidea
11. Sinus sphenoidalis
12. Sinus frontalis, kaudomedialer Rand – *caudomedial border*
13. Canalis opticus
14. Fissura orbitalis
15. Foramen rotundum
16. Foramen ovale
17. Hamulus pterygoideus
18. Cavum cranii, rostrale Wand – *rostral border*
19. Os frontale, Processus zygomaticus
20. Ostium tympanicum tubae auditivae
21. Porus acusticus externus
22. Meatus acusticus externus cartilagineus
23. Ossicula auditus
24. Foramen jugulare
25. Dorsum sellae turcicae
26. Os temporale, Bulla tympanica
27. Os temporale, Pars petrosa
28. Tentorium cerebelli osseum
29. Os temporale, Processus retrotympanicus
30. Fossa condylaris ventralis
31. Condylus occipitalis
32. Foramen magnum, ventraler Rand – *ventral border*
33. Crista nuchae, lateral Crista temporalis
34. Os temporale, Processus zygomaticus

C Mandibula
35. Processus condylaris
36. Processus coronoideus
37. Processus angularis
38. Corpus mandibulae

Ca Dens caninus

J Dentes incisivi

M₁ Dens molaris I

D Atlas
39. Arcus ventralis, kranialer Rand – *cranial border*
40. Arcus ventralis, kaudaler Rand – *caudal border*
41. Arcus dorsalis, kaudaler Rand – *caudal border*
42. Foramen transversarium
43. Ala atlantis
44. Incisura alaris
45. Fovea articularis caudalis

E Axis
46. Dens
47. Processus articularis cranialis
48. Processus spinosus
49. Incisura vertebralis cranialis
50. Pediculus arcus vertebrae
51. Extremitas caudalis
52. Processus transversus

F C III

G Os hyoideum

1 Kopf – Head

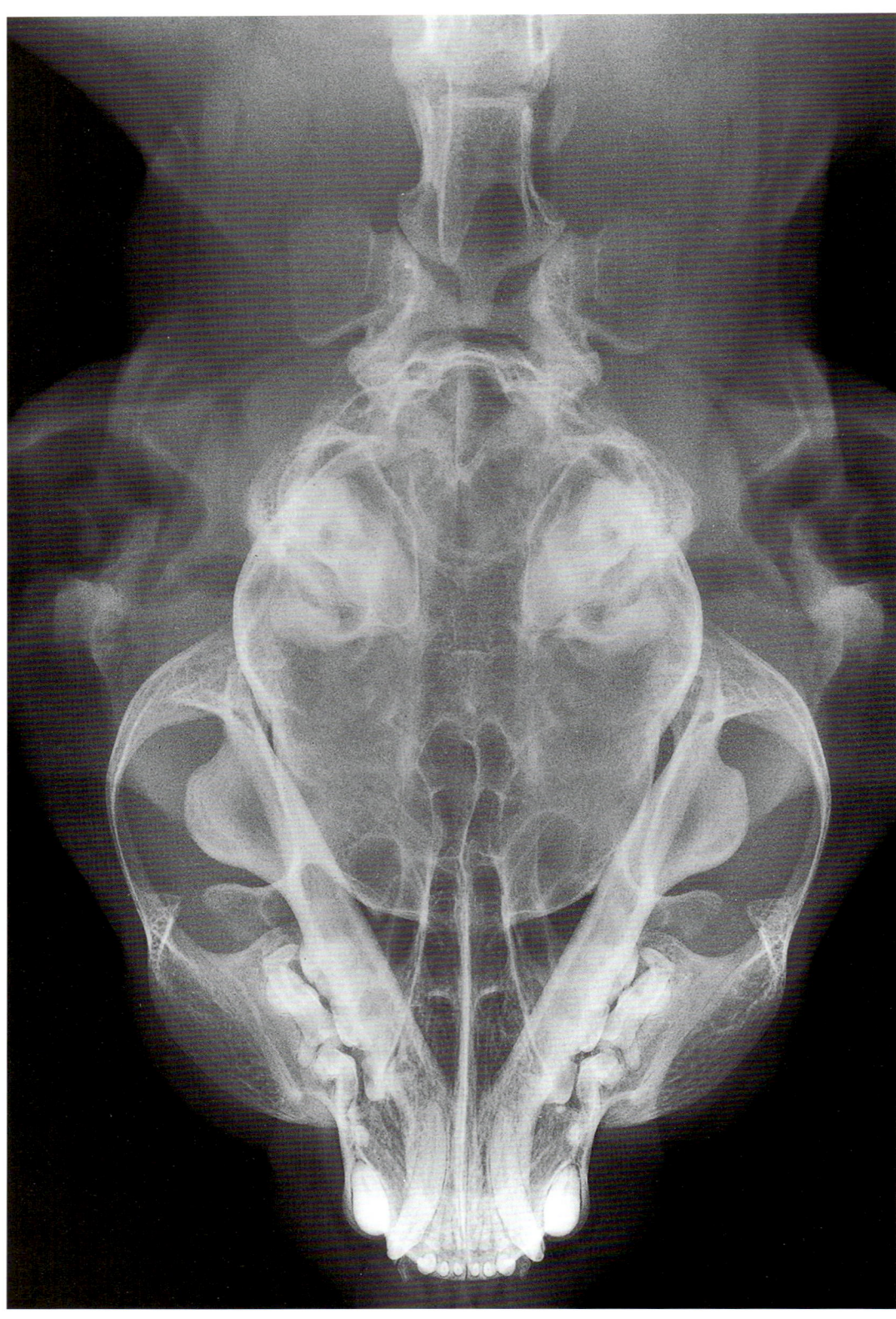

Abb. 1.3 Kopf, dorso-ventral,
Katze
(Ausschnitt aus 13 × 18 cm)

Fig. 1.3 Head, dorso-ventral,
Cat
(section of 13 × 18 cm)

■ **Ziel**
Symmetrische Darstellung der Kopfknochen und der Schädelhöhle.

■ **Zentralstrahl**
Senkrecht zur Kassette, auf die Medianlinie des Kopfes in Höhe der temporalen Augenwinkel.

■ **Beachte**
Die Kehlränder des Unterkiefers in gleicher Höhe zur Kassette. Schon eine geringe Verkantung verursacht erhebliche Verzeichnungen und Überlagerungen. Kassette durch Unterlegen eines etwa 3 cm hohen Holzbrettes anheben.

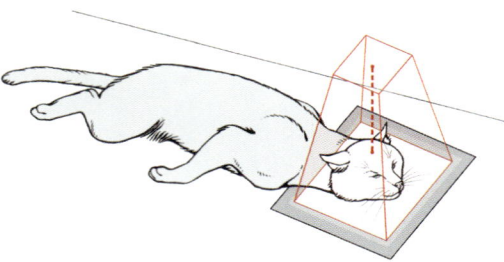

Abb. 1.3 Lagerung zur Aufnahme des Kopfes. Dorso-ventral.

Fig. 1.3 Positioning of head. Dorso-ventral.

■ *Objective*
To obtain a symmetric dorso-ventral radiographic image of the cranial cavity.

■ *Central ray of the primary beam*
Direct the x-ray beam perpendicular to the cassette, with the central ray centered on the median plane at the level of the temporal angle of the eye.

■ *Notice*
Position the head with the ventral borders of the mandibles at the same level. Even a slight tilting or rotation of the head causes considerable distortion and superimposition. Raise the cassette with a wooden board (approximately 1 inch thick).

1.3 Kopf – Head ■ dorso-ventral

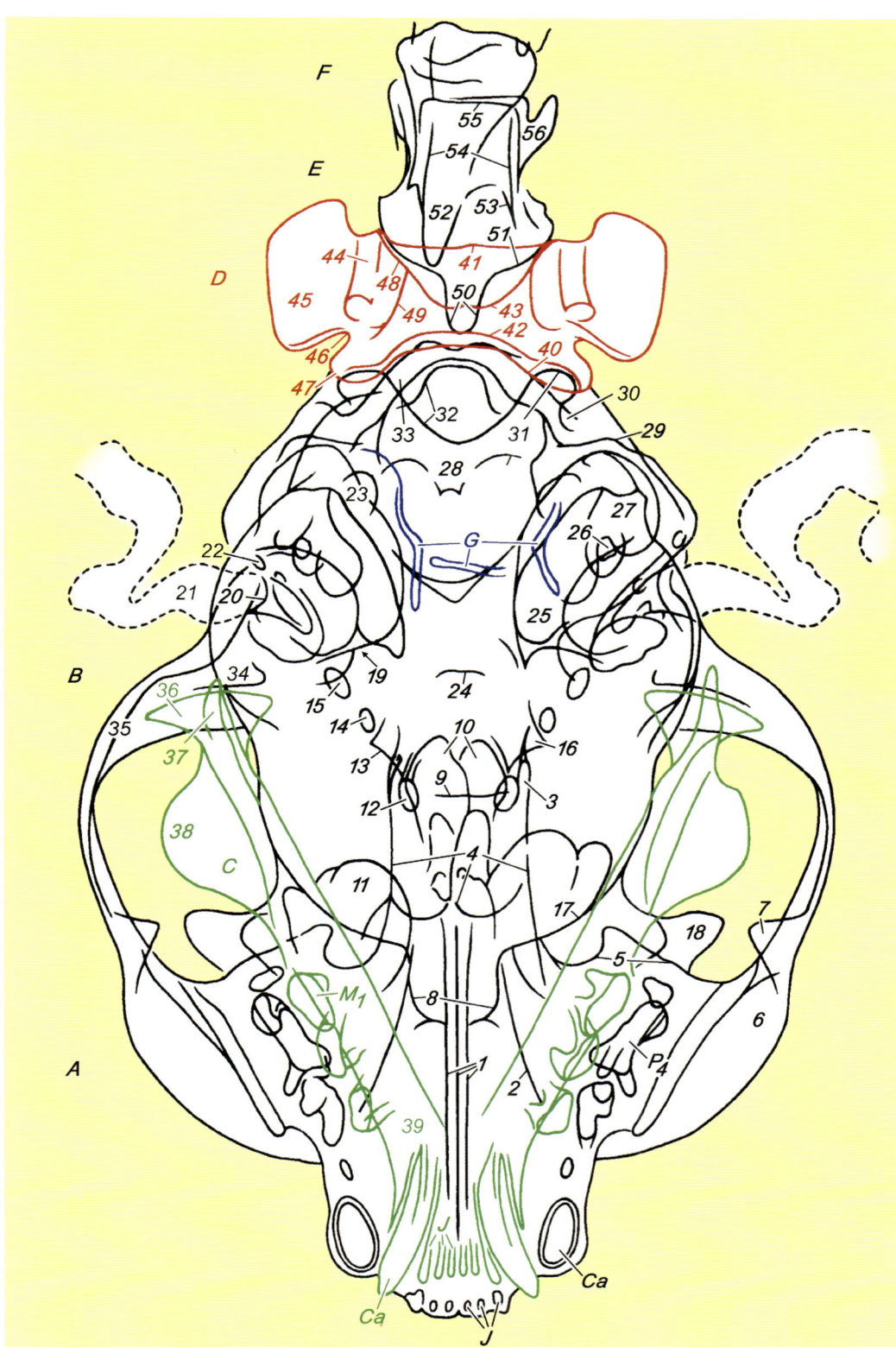

15	Foramen ovale
16	Hamulus pterygoideus
17	Cavum cranii, rostrale Wand – *rostral border*
18	Os frontale, Processus zygomaticus
19	Os temporale, Ostium tympanicum tubae auditivae
20	Os temporale, Porus acusticus externus
21	Meatus acusticus externus cartilagineus
22	Os temporale, Foramen stylomastoideum
23	Foramen jugulare
24	Dorsum sellae turcicae
25	Os temporale, Bulla tympanica
26	Os temporale, Porus acusticus internus
27	Os temporale, Pars petrosa
28	Tentorium cerebelli osseum
29	Os temporale, Processus retrotympanicus
30	Fossa condylaris ventralis
31	Condylus occipitalis
32	Foramen magnum
33	Crista nuchae, lateral Crista temporalis
34	Processus retroarticularis
35	Os temporale, Processus zygomaticus

C Mandibula
- **36** Processus condylaris
- **37** Processus angularis
- **38** Processus coronoideus
- **39** Corpus mandibulae

J Dentes incisivi

Ca Dens caninus

M₁ Dens molaris I

D Atlas
- **40** Arcus dorsalis, kranialer Rand – *cranial border*
- **41** Arcus dorsalis, kaudaler Rand – *caudal border*
- **42** Arcus ventralis, kranialer Rand – *cranial border*
- **43** Arcus ventralis, kaudaler Rand – *caudal border*
- **44** Foramen transversarium
- **45** Ala atlantis
- **46** Incisura alaris
- **47** Fovea articularis cranialis
- **48** Fovea articularis caudalis
- **49** Foramen vertebrale, seitliche Begrenzung – *lateral border*

E Axis
- **50** Dens
- **51** Processus articularis cranialis
- **52** Processus spinosus
- **53** Incisura vertebralis cranialis
- **54** Foramen vertebrale, seitliche Begrenzung – *lateral border*
- **55** Extremitas caudalis
- **56** Processus transversus

F C III

G Anteile des Os hyoideum – *parts of Os hyoideum*

A Ossa faciei
1. Sutura palatina mediana et Vomer
2. Cavum nasi, Wand – *wall*
3. Choana, Wand – *wall*
4. Choana et Spina nasalis caudalis
5. Os maxillare, kaudaler Rand – *caudal border*
6. Os zygomaticum, Processus temporalis
7. Os zygomaticum, Processus frontalis

J Dentes incisivi

Ca Dens caninus
P₄ Dens praemolaris IV

B Ossa cranii
8. Fossa ethmoidalis
9. Crista orbitosphenoidea
10. Sinus sphenoidalis
11. Sinus frontalis
12. Canalis opticus
13. Fissura orbitalis
14. Foramen rotundum

1 Kopf – Head

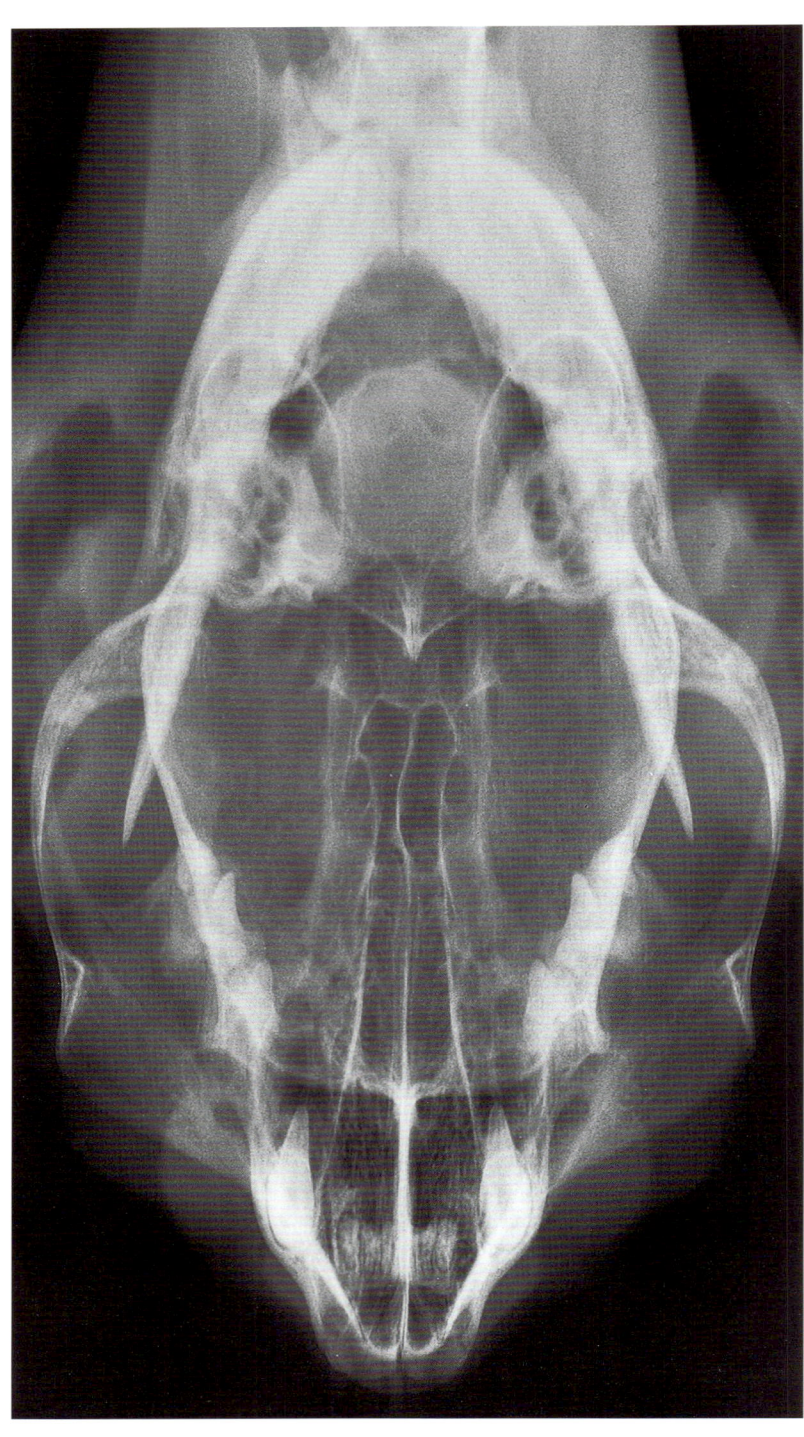

Abb. 1.4 Oberkiefer bei geöffneter Mundhöhle, ventro-dorsal, Schrägprojektion,
Katze
(Ausschnitt aus 13 × 18 cm)

Fig. 1.4 Upper jaw with open mouth, ventro-dorsal, oblique,
Cat
(section of 13 × 18 cm)

■ **Ziel**
Aufnahme des Oberkiefers ohne Überlagerung durch den Unterkiefer.

■ **Zentralstrahl**
In die weit geöffnete Mundhöhle, im Winkel von 45° auf die Raphe palati in Höhe des P_3.

■ **Beachte**
Stirn und Nasenrücken möglichst plan auf die Kassette, Mundspalte weit geöffnet. Die Öffnung der Kiefergelenke kann durch zwei Bänder fixiert werden.

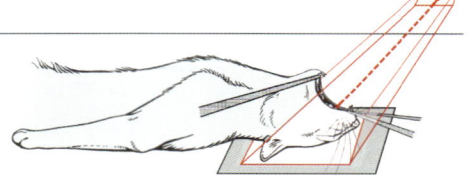

Abb. 1.4 Lagerung zur Aufnahme des Oberkiefers bei geöffneter Mundspalte. Ventro-dorsal. Schrägprojektion.

Fig. 1.4 Positioning of the upper jaw with open mouth. Ventro-dorsal. Oblique.

■ *Objective*
To image the upper jaw without superimposition by the lower jaw.

■ *Central ray of the primary beam*
The x-ray beam and the raphe palati create an angle of 45°, centered at the level of P_3.

■ *Notice*
Align the forehead and dorsum nasi as close as possible to the cassette, open the mouth wide. Opening of the temporo-mandibular joints is fixed by two straps.

1.4 Oberkiefer – Upper jaw ■ ventro-dorsal

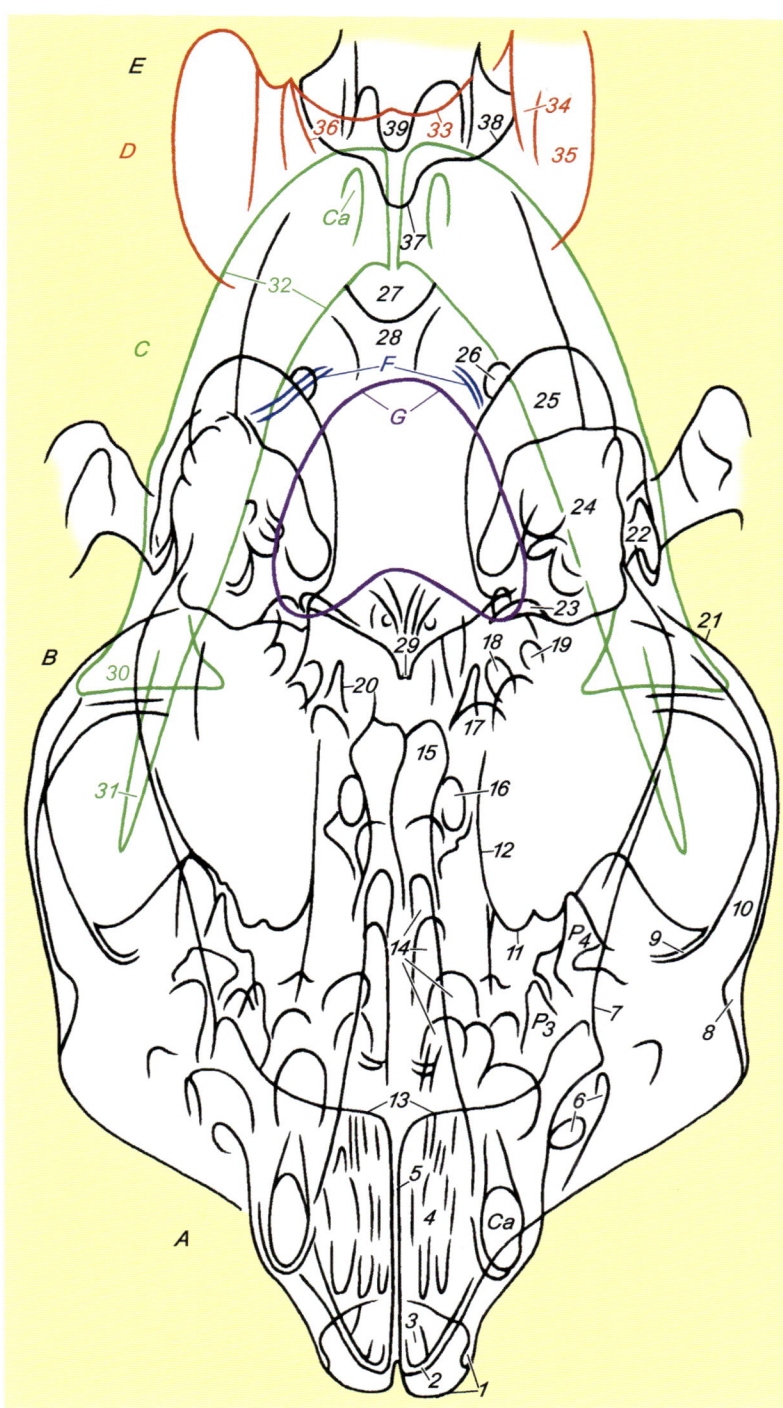

A Ossa faciei
1. Os nasale
2. Os incisivum, Corpus, rostraler Rand – *rostral border*
3. Fissura palatina
4. Cavum nasi et Os conchae nasalis ventralis
5. Septum nasi
6. Foramen et Canalis infraorbitalis
7. Os maxillare, Processus alveolaris
8. Os zygomaticum
9. Sutura zygomaticomaxillaris
10. Os zygomaticum, Processus temporalis
11. Os palatinum, Lamina horizontalis
12. Choanae, lateraler Rand – *lateral border*

Ca Dens caninus
P_3 Dens praemolaris III
P_4 Dens praemolaris IV

B Ossa cranii
13. Cavum cranii, rostrale Wand – *rostral border*
14. Os ethmoidale, Endoturbinalia
15. Sinus sphenoidalis
16. Foramen opticum
17. Fissura orbitalis
18. Foramen rotundum
19. Foramen ovale
20. Hamulus pterygoideus
21. Os temporale, Processus zygomaticus
22. Os temporale, Porus acusticus externus
23. Os temporale, Ostium tympanicum tubae auditivae
24. Os temporale, Pars petrosa
25. Os temporale, Bulla tympanica
26. Foramen jugulare
27. Foramen magnum
28. Os occipitale, Pars basilaris
29. Dorsum sellae turcicae

C Mandibula
30. Processus condylaris
31. Processus coronoideus
32. Corpus mandibulae

Ca Dens caninus

D Atlas
33. Arcus ventralis, kaudaler Rand – *caudal border*
34. Foramen transversarium
35. Ala atlantis
36. Fovea articularis caudalis

E Axis
37. Dens
38. Processus articularis cranialis
39. Processus spinosus

F Anteile des Os hyoideum – *parts of Os hyoideum*

G Lingua

1 Kopf – Head

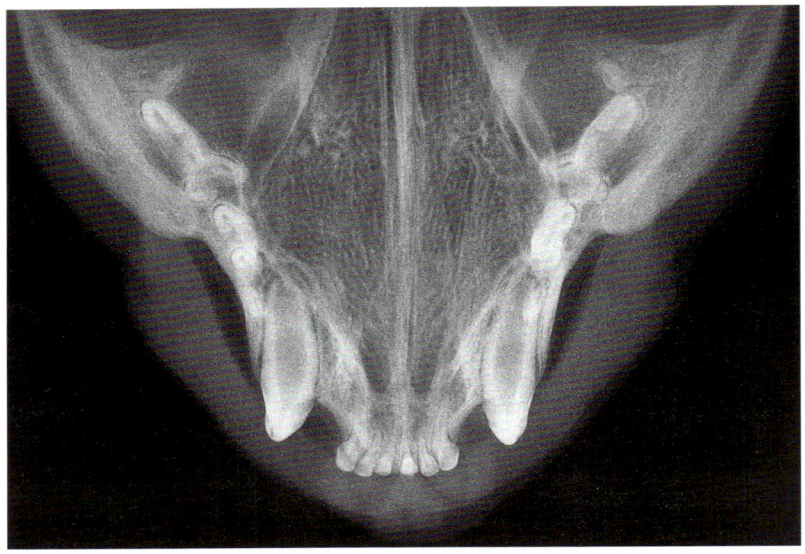

**Abb. 1.5 Oberkiefer
(Kassette in der Mundhöhle),
dorso-ventral,**
Katze

*Fig. 1.5 Upper jaw
(cassette in oral cavity),
dorso-ventral,*
Cat

■ **Ziel**
Darstellung der Oberkieferzähne und der Nasenhöhle.

■ **Zentralstrahl**
Senkrecht zur Kassette, auf die Medianlinie des Kopfes in Höhe des P_3.

■ **Beachte**
Mundspalte nach Einlegen der Kassette vorsichtig schließen.
Verkanten des Kopfes durch Fixierung vermeiden.
Kopf durch Unterlegen z. B. eines Holzbrettes oder eines Schaumgummikeils anheben.

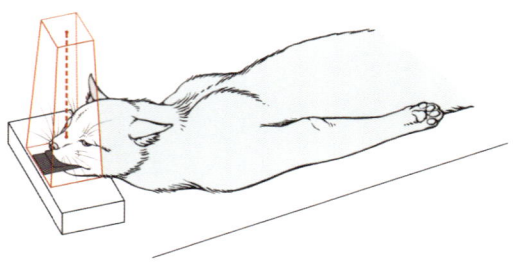

Abb. 1.5 Lagerung zur Aufnahme des Oberkiefers. Dorso-ventral. Kassette in die Mundhöhle eingelegt.

Fig. 1.5 Positioning of upper jaw. Dorso-ventral. Cassette placed in oral cavity.

■ *Objective*
To image the superior teeth and the nasal cavity.

■ *Central ray of the primary beam*
Direct the x-ray beam perpendicular to the cassette, centered at the level of P_3.

■ *Notice*
Use an intraoral cassette and close the mouth carefully.
Fix the head symmetrically to prevent tilting.
Raise the head with a wooden board or a foam rubber wedge.

1.5 Oberkiefer – Upper jaw ■ dorso-ventral

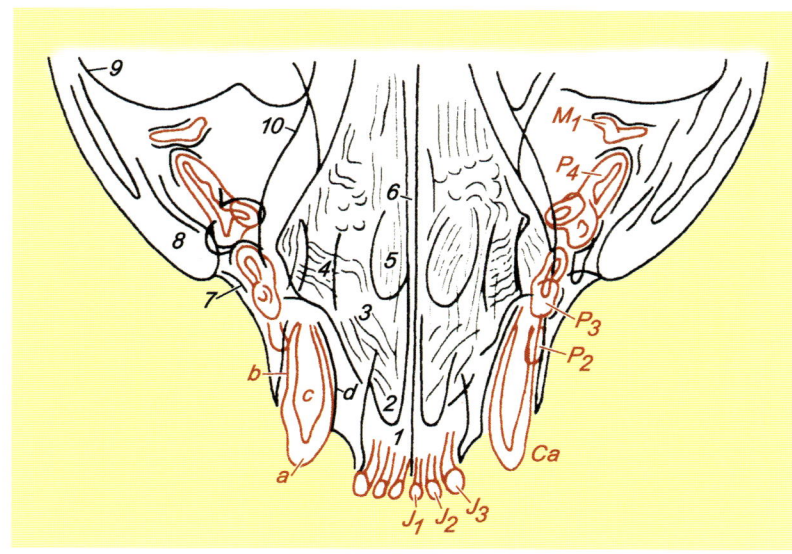

1 Os incisivum, Corpus
2 Fissura palatina
3 Cavum nasi et Conchae nasales
4 Recessus maxillaris
5 Sinus frontalis, rostraler Teil – *rostral part*
6 Septum nasi
7 Foramen infraorbitale
8 Os maxillare et Os zygomaticum, Corpus
9 Arcus zygomaticus
10 Orbitawand, mediale Wand – *medial border*

J_1–J_3   Dentes incisivi I – III

Ca Dens caninus

P_2–P_4   Dentes praemolares II – IV

M_1 Dens molaris I

a   Corona dentis (Ca)

b   Radix dentis

c   Cavum dentis

d   Alveolus dentalis (maxillae)

1 Kopf – Head

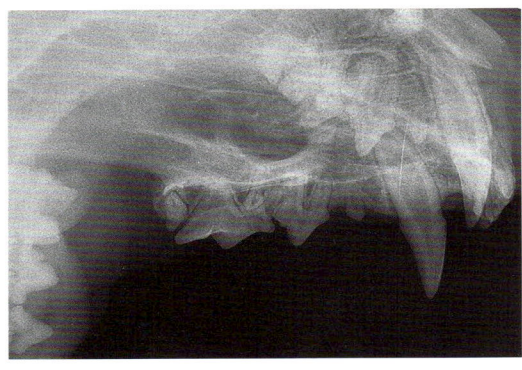 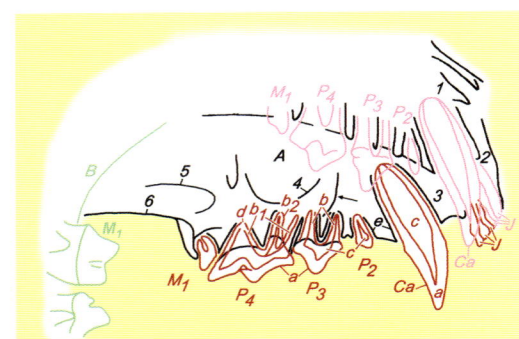

Abb. 1.6 Oberkiefer bei geöffneter Mundhöhle, medio-lateral, Schräglagerung,
Katze
(Ausschnitt aus 9 × 12 cm)

Fig. 1.6 Upper jaw with open mouth, medio-lateral, oblique positioning,
Cat
(section of 9 × 12 cm)

A Os faciei
1 Os nasale
2 Corpus ossis incisivi
3 Os incisivum, Processus alveolaris
4 Recessus maxillaris
5 Choanenrand – *border of Choana*
6 Arcus zygomaticus, Ventralrand – *ventral border*

Pfeil kennzeichnet rostralen Rand des Foramen infraorbitale – *arrow indicates the rostral border of Foramen infraorbitale*

B Mandibula, Ramus, plattenfern – *next to the tube*

M_1 Dens molaris I

J Dentes incisivi I– III

Ca Dens caninus

P_2–P_4 Dentes praemolares II– IV

M_1 Dens molaris I

a Corona dentis (Ca)

b Radix dentis (P_3, P_4)

b_1 Radices buccales (P_3, P_4)

b_2 Radix lingualis (P_4)

c Cavum dentis (Ca, P_2, P_3)

d Foramen apicis dentis (P_4)

e Alveolus dentalis (maxillae)

■ **Ziel**
Aufnahme einer Oberkieferseite ohne Überlagerung.

■ **Zentralstrahl**
Senkrecht zur Kassette in Höhe des Alveolarrandes von P_3.

■ **Beachte**
Seitenlagerung oder halbe Rückenlagerung der Katze, Mundspalte weit geöffnet. Die Öffnung der Kiefer kann durch zwei Bänder fixiert werden.
Den Kopf durch Unterlegen eines Schaumgummikeils so drehen, dass der harte Gaumen einen Winkel von 45° zur Kassette bildet.

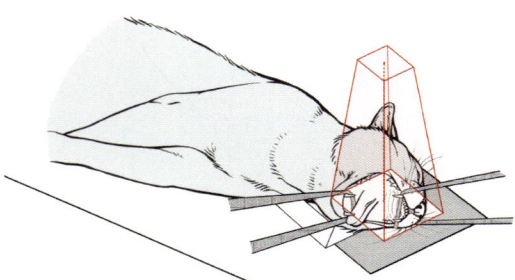

Abb. 1.6 Schräglagerung zur Aufnahme des Oberkiefers bei geöffneter Mundhöhle. Medio-lateral.

Fig. 1.6 Oblique positioning of upper jaw with open mouth. Medio-lateral.

■ *Objective*
To image one upper jaw without superimposition.

■ *Central ray of the primary beam*
Direct the x-ray beam perpendicular to the cassette, centered at the level of P_3.

■ *Notice*
Lateral recumbency or half dorsal positioning of the cat, open the mouth wide. Opening of the temporo-mandibular joints is fixed by two straps.
Use a foam rubber wedge to rotate the head so that the hard palate and the cassette form an angle of 45°.

1.7 Unterkiefer – Lower jaw ■ medio-lateral

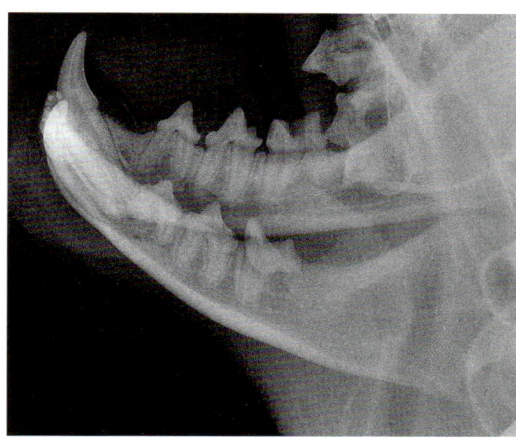
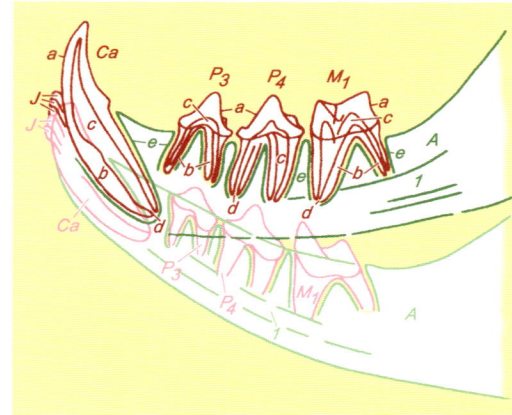

Abb. 1.7 Unterkiefer bei geöffneter Mundhöhle, medio-lateral, Schräglagerung,
Katze
(Ausschnitt aus 9 × 12 cm)

*Fig. 1.7 Lower jaw with open mouth, medio-lateral, oblique positioning,
Cat
(section of 9 × 12 cm)*

A Mandibula, Corpus
   1 Canalis mandibulae

J Dentes incisivi I–III

Ca Dens caninus

P_3 Dens praemolaris III

P_4 Dens praemolaris IV

M_1 Dens molaris I

a Corona dentis (Ca, P_3, P_4, M_1)

b Radix dentis (Ca, P_3, M_1)

c Cavum dentis (Ca, P_3, P_4, M_1)

d Foramen apicis dentis (Ca, P_4, M_1)

e Alveolus dentalis (mandibulae)

■ Ziel
Aufnahme einer Unterkieferseite ohne Überlagerung.

Zentralstrahl
Senkrecht zur Kassette in Höhe des Alveolarrandes von P_4.

■ Beachte
Bauchlage der Katze. Das Öffnen der Mundspalte gelingt mit 2 Bändern um die Canini des Unter- bzw. Oberkiefers. Unterlegen der gekippten Kopfseite (45°) durch einen fixierten Schaumgummikeil.

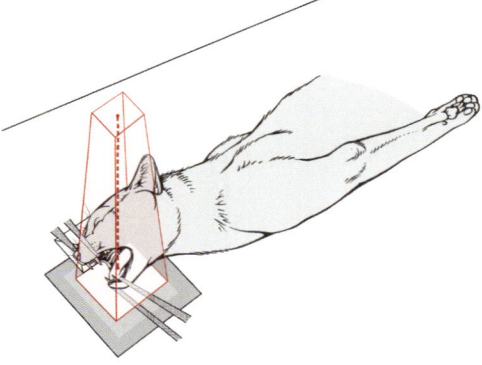

Abb. 1.7 Schräglagerung zur Aufnahme des Unterkiefers bei geöffneter Mundspalte. Medio-lateral.

Fig. 1.7 Oblique positioning of lower jaw with open mouth. Medio-lateral.

■ *Objective*
To image one lower jaw without superimposition.

Central ray of the primary beam
Direct the x-ray beam perpendicular to the cassette, centered at the level of P_4.

■ *Notice*
Abdominal recumbency of the cat. Opening of the mouth by two straps placed over the upper or lower canini.
Use a foam rubber wedge to tilt the head (by 45°).

1 Kopf – Head

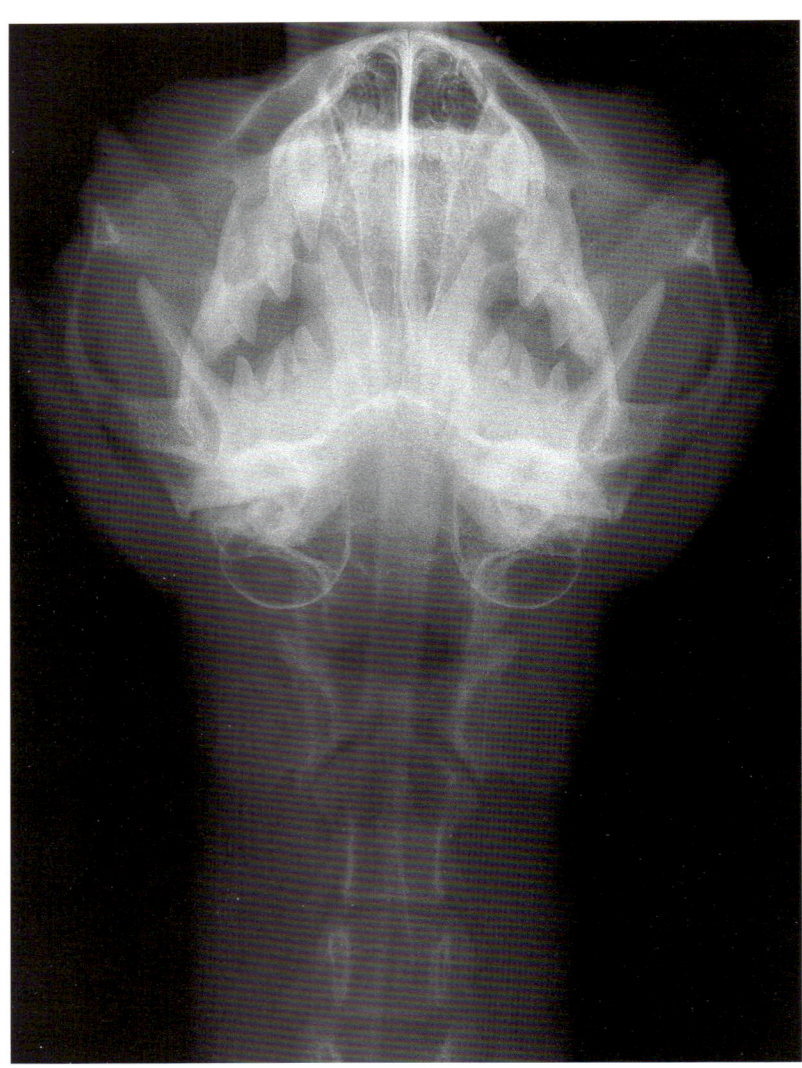

Abb. 1.8 Bulla tympanica, ventro-dorsal, Katze

Fig. 1.8 Bulla tympanica, ventro-dorsal, Cat

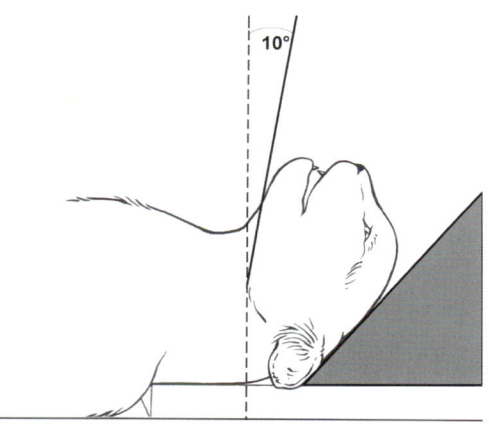

■ **Ziel**
Überlagerungsfreie, symmetrische Aufnahme der Bullae tympanicae.

■ **Zentralstrahl**
Senkrecht zur Kassette auf das Kinn.

■ **Beachte**
Durch Unterlegen eines steilen Schaumgummikeiles an der Stirn der Katze soll ein Winkel von 10° zur Senkrechten am Ventralrand des Corpus mandibulae erreicht werden.

Abb. 1.8 Lagerung zur Aufnahme der Bulla tympanica. Ventro-dorsal.
(nach HOFER et al., 1999)

Fig. 1.8 Positioning of Bulla tympanica. Ventro-dorsal.
(after HOFER et al., 1999)

■ *Objective*
To image symmetrically the tympanic bullae without superimposition.

■ *Central ray of the primary beam*
Direct the x-ray beam perpendicular to the cassette, centered at the level of the mentum.

■ *Notice*
Use a steep foam rubber wedge at the frontal plane of the head to achieve an angle of 10° to the vertical plane at the ventral borders of the mandibles.

1.8 Bulla tympanica – Bulla tympanica ■ ventro-dorsal

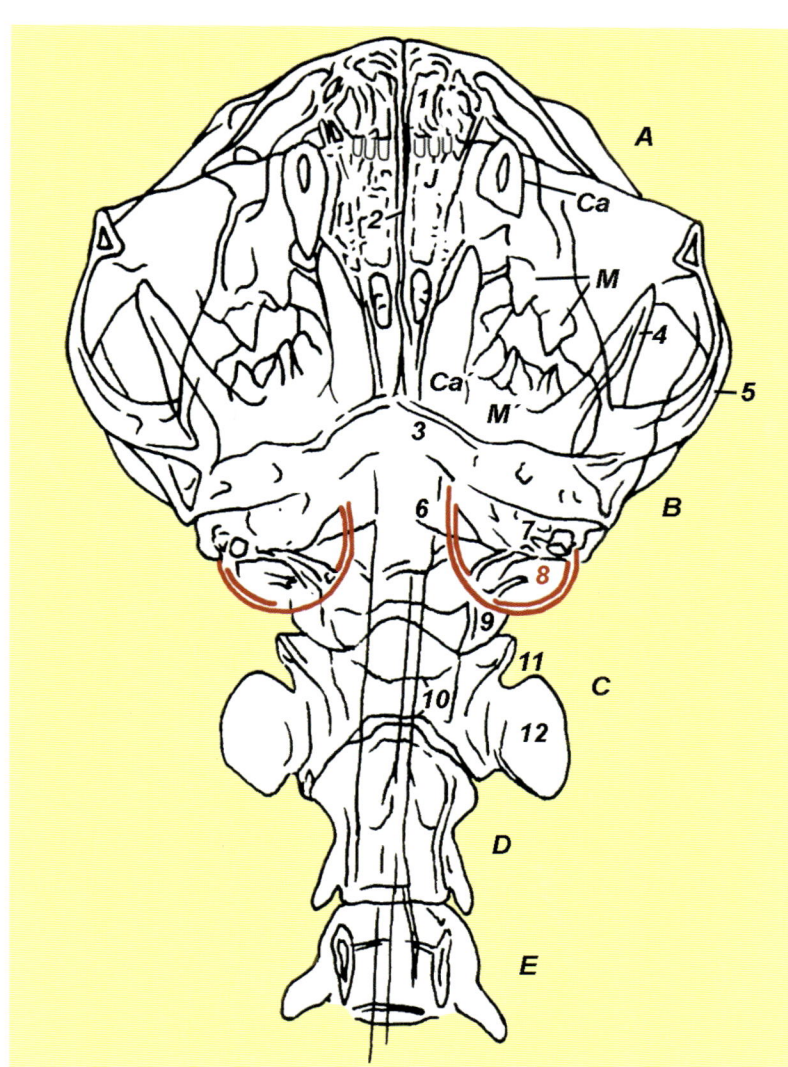

A Ossa faciei

- J   Incisivi (maxillar)
- Ca Caninus
- Ca´ Caninus (mandibular)
- M Molares (maxillar)
- M´ Molares (mandibular)
  - 1   Conchae nasales
  - 2   Vomer
  - 3   Corpus mandibulae
  - 4   Processus condylaris
  - 5   Arcus zygomaticus

B Ossa cranii

- 6   Crista nuchae
- 7   Porus acusticus externus
- **8   Bulla tympanica**
- 9   Condylus occipitalis

C Atlas

- 10 Arcus ventralis
- 11 Incisura alaris
- 12 Ala atlantis

D Axis

E CIII

29

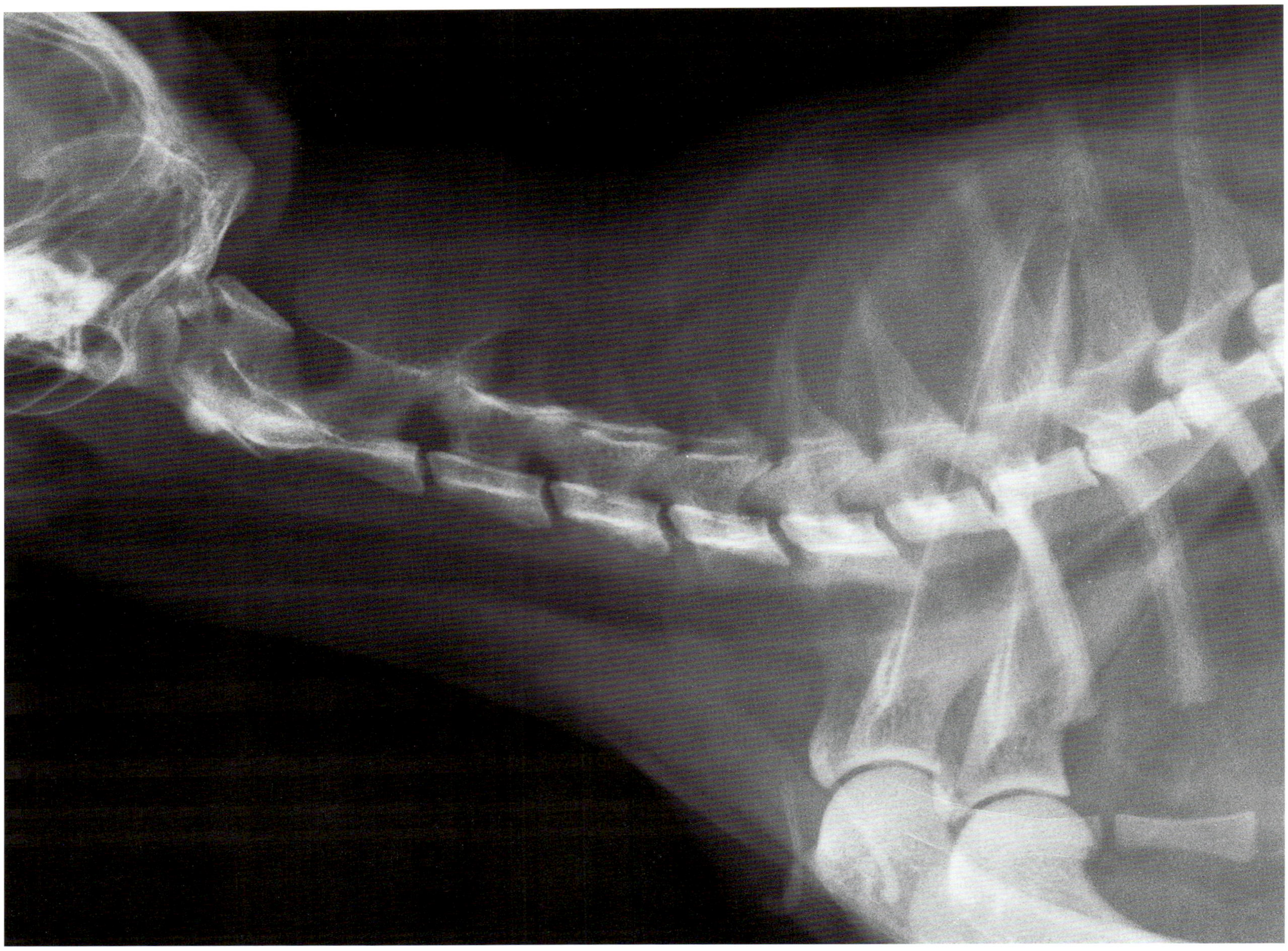

2 Wirbelsäule – Vertebral column

Abb. 2.1 Halswirbelsäule, latero-lateral,
Katze
(Ausschnitt aus 13 × 18 cm)

Fig. 2.1 Cervical vertebral column, latero-lateral,
Cat
(section of 13 × 18 cm)

■ **Ziel**
Darstellung der gestreckten Halswirbelsäule ohne Verkantung.

■ **Zentralstrahl**
Senkrecht zur Kassette, in Höhe des Ventralrandes des 4. Halswirbels.

■ **Beachte**
Medianebene des Kopfes und des Rumpfes parallel zur Kassette. Hierbei helfen Schaumgummikeile unter der rostralen Kopfhälfte, dem Hals und der Schulter der unten liegenden, kaudal gelagerten Schultergliedmaße.
Die Extremitäten und der Schwanz sollten kaudal gestreckt werden.

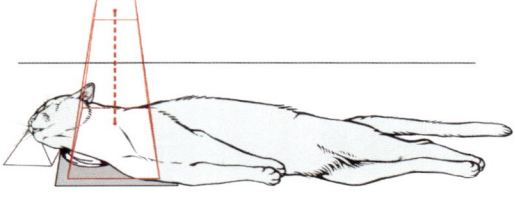

Abb. 2.1 Lagerung zur Aufnahme der Halswirbelsäule. Latero-lateral.

Fig. 2.1 Positioning of cervical vertebral column. Latero-lateral.

■ *Objective*
To image the extended cervical spine without rotation and sagging of the vertebral column.

■ *Central ray of the primary beam*
Direct the x-ray beam perpendicular to the cassette, centered on the ventral edge of C4.

■ *Notice*
Align the median plane of the head and body parallel to the cassette, support the rostral part of head, neck and dependent shoulder with foam rubber wedges.
The limbs and the tail should be extended caudally.

2.1 Halswirbelsäule – Cervical vertebral column ■ latero-lateral

A Os occipitale
1. Crista sagittalis externa
2. Crista nuchae
3. Squama occipitalis
4. Foramen magnum, dorsaler Rand – *dorsal border*
5. Condylus occipitalis
6. Os occipitale, Pars basilaris
7. Bulla tympanica

B Atlas
8. Arcus dorsalis
9. Arcus ventralis
10. Fovea articularis cranialis
11. Ala atlantis
12. Foramen vertebrale laterale
13. Gefäßloch – *vascular foramen*

C Axis
14. Dens
15. Corpus vertebrae
16. Processus articularis cranialis
17. Foramen vertebrale, ventrale bzw. dorsale Begrenzung – *ventral and dorsal border respectively*
18. Incisura vertebralis cranialis
19. Processus spinosus
20. Processus articularis caudalis
21. Incisura vertebralis caudalis
22. Processus transversus
23. Foramen transversarium
24. Facies terminalis caudalis

D C III

E C IV (15–22, 24, siehe – *see* C, Axis)
25. Facies terminalis cranialis
26. Tuberculum ventrale

F C V

G C VI (15–22, 24, siehe – *see* C, Axis; E, C IV)
26. Lamina ventralis

H C VII

J T I (15–22, 25, siehe – *see* C, Axis; E, C IV)

K Os costale I

L Sternum

M Scapula
27. Spina scapulae
28. Acromion
29. Tuberculum supraglenoidale
30. Tuberculum infraglenoidale

N Clavicula

O Humerus

P Trachea

2 Wirbelsäule – Vertebral column

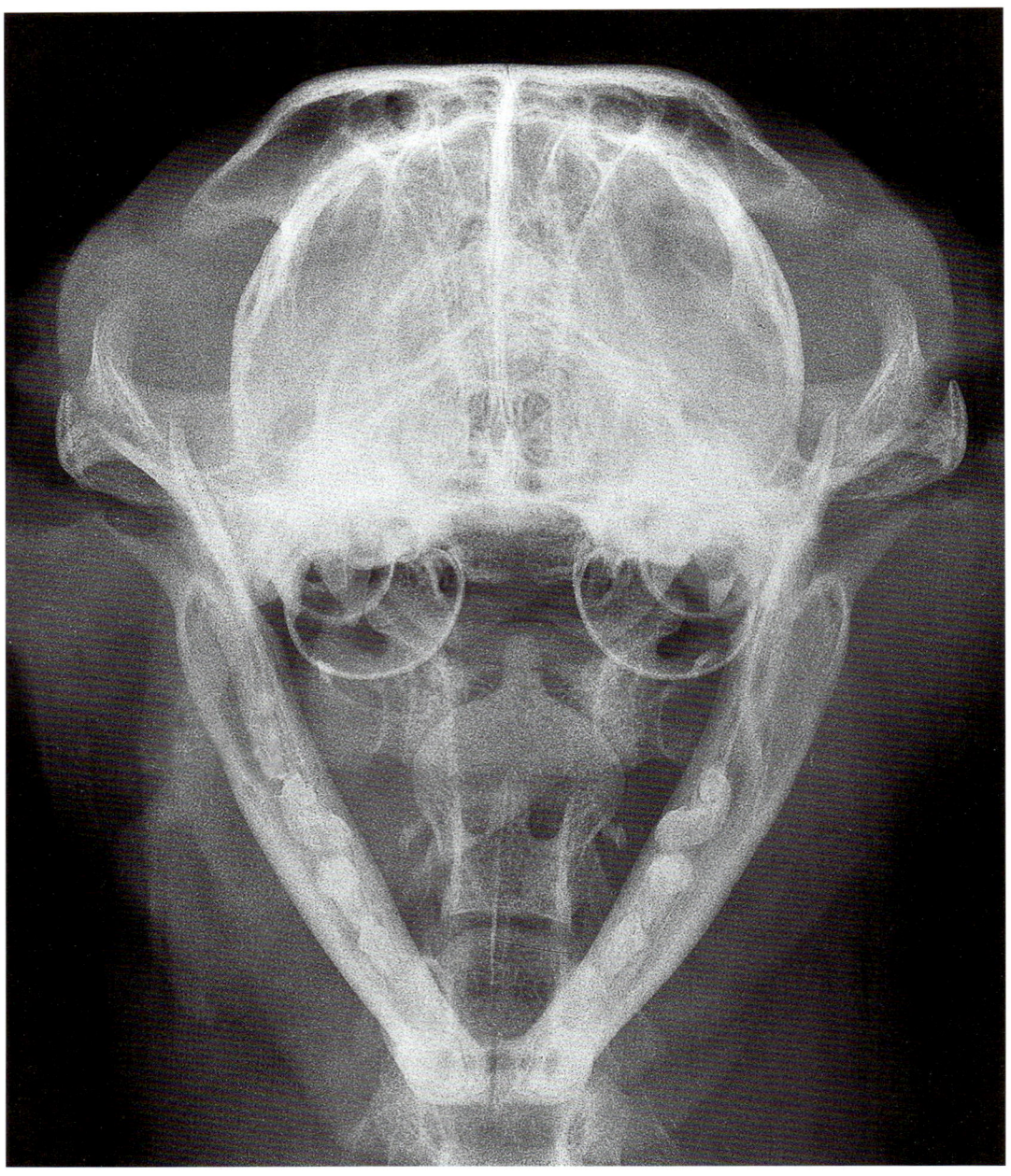

Abb. 2.2 1. und 2. Halswirbel durch die geöffnete Mundhöhle, rostro-kaudal,
Katze
(Ausschnitt aus 13 × 18 cm)

Fig. 2.2 1st and 2nd cervical vertebrae through the open mouth, rostro-caudal,
Katze
(section of 13 × 18 cm)

■ **Ziel**
Nicht überlagerte Darstellung von Atlas und Axis (Dens).

■ **Zentralstrahl**
Durch die geöffnete Mundhöhle, senkrecht auf die Medianebene in Höhe des Zungengrundes.

■ **Beachte**
Kopf und Rumpf exakt senkrecht zur Kassette fixiert.
Die geöffnete Mundhöhle ist mit 2 Bändern so zu lagern, dass der harte Gaumen etwa im Winkel von 80° zur Kassette steht.
(Bei der narkotisierten Katze ist die Zunge gerade vorzulagern.)

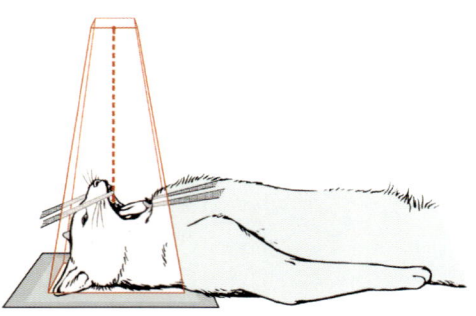

Abb. 2.2 Lagerung zur Aufnahme des 1. und 2. Halswirbels durch die geöffnete Mundhöhle. Rostro-kaudal.

Fig. 2.2 Positioning of 1st and 2nd cervical vertebrae through the open mouth. Rostro-caudal.

■ *Objective*
To image the atlas and axis (dens) without superimposition.

■ *Central ray of the primary beam*
Direct the x-ray beam through the opened mouth, centered along the median plane, at the level of the tongue's root.

■ *Notice*
Align head and body exactly perpendicular to the cassette.
Opening of the mouth by two straps placed over the upper or lower incisor teeth. The hard palate should have an angle of about 80° to the cassette.
(Pull the tongue of the anesthetized cat rostrally.)

2.2 1. und 2. Halswirbel – 1st and 2nd cervical vertebrae ■ rostro-kaudal – rostro-caudal

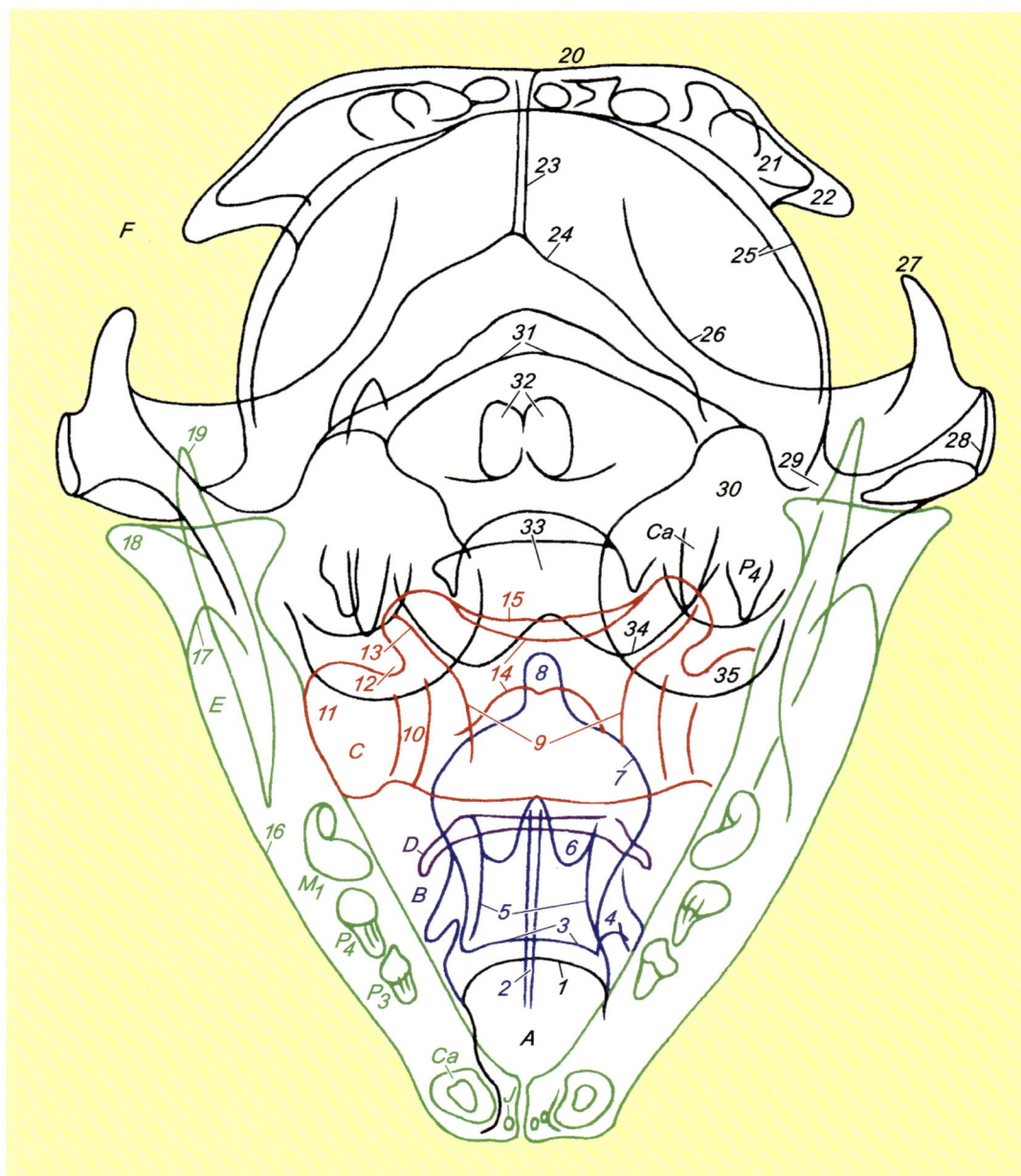

A C III
1 Facies terminalis cranialis

B Axis
2 Processus spinosus
3 Facies terminalis caudalis
4 Processus transversus
5 Foramen vertebrale
6 Incisura vertebralis cranialis
7 Processus articularis cranialis
8 Dens

C Atlas
9 Foramen vertebrale
10 Foramen transversarium
11 Ala atlantis
12 Incisura alaris
13 Fovea articularis cranialis
14 Arcus ventralis
15 Arcus dorsalis, kranialer Rand – *cranial border*

D Os hyoideum

E Mandibula
16 Corpus mandibulae
17 Angulus mandibulae
18 Processus condylaris
19 Processus coronoideus

J Dens incisivus

Ca Dens caninus

P₃ Dens praemolaris III

P₄ Dens praemolaris IV

M₁ Dens molaris I

F Ossa cranii et faciei
20 Os frontale, Facies externa
21 Sinus frontalis
22 Os frontale, Processus zygomaticus
23 Crista sagittalis externa
24 Crista nuchae
25 Cavum cranii, laterale Wand – *lateral wall*
26 Orbita, mediale Wand – *medial wall*
27 Os zygomaticum, Processus frontalis
28 Arcus zygomaticus
29 Tuberculum articulare
30 Os temporale, Partes petrosa et tympanica
31 Tentorium cerebelli osseum
32 Os ethmoidale, Lamina cribosa
33 Foramen magnum
34 Condylus occipitalis
35 Os temporale, Bulla tympanica

Ca Dens caninus

P₄ Dens praemolaris IV

2 Wirbelsäule – Vertebral column

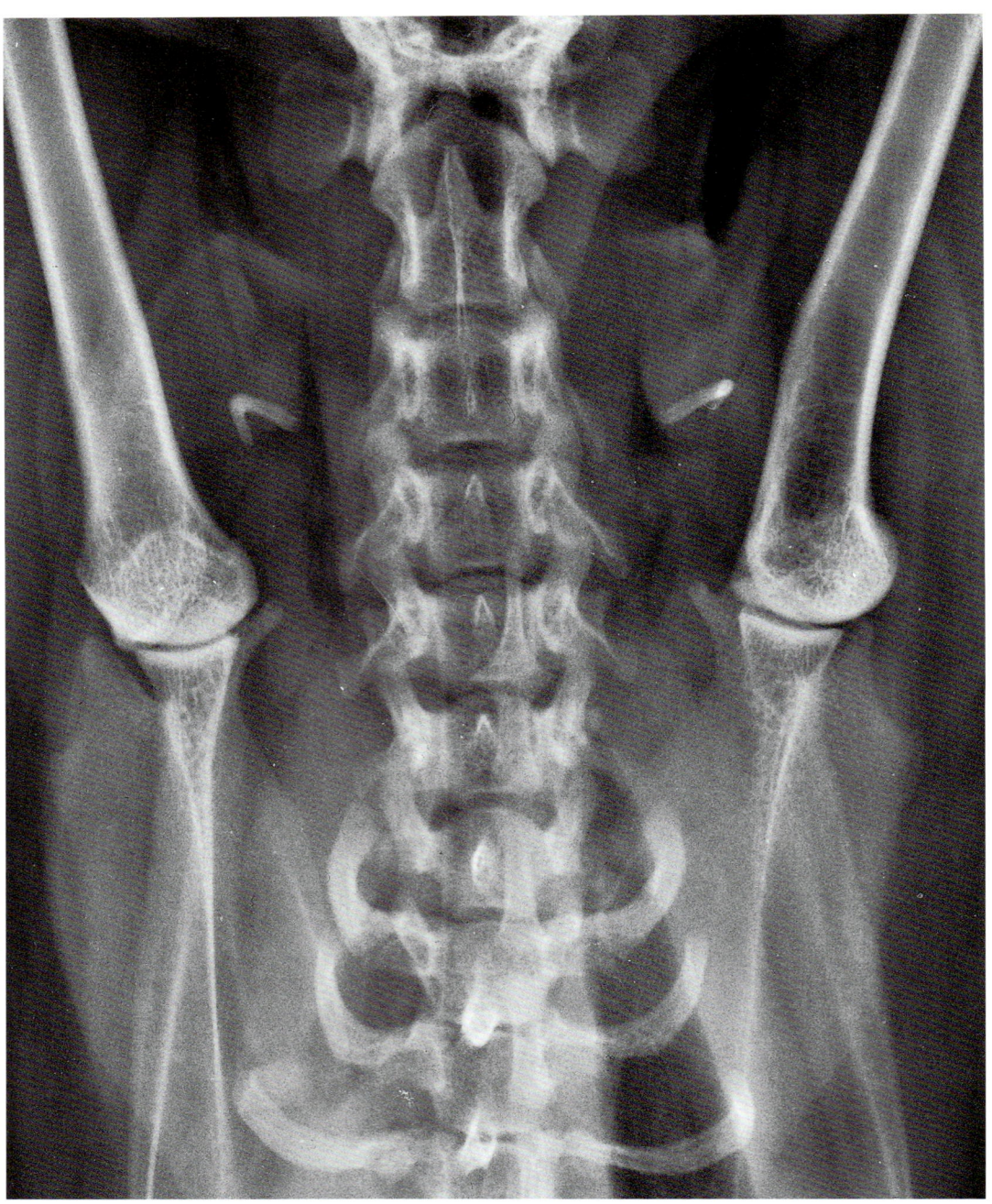

**Abb. 2.3 Halswirbelsäule,
ventro-dorsal,**
Katze
(Ausschnitt aus 18 × 24 cm)

*Fig. 2.3 Cervical vertebral column,
ventro-dorsal,*
Cat
(section of 18 × 24 cm)

■ **Ziel**
Darstellung der gestreckten, symmetrischen Halswirbel.

■ **Zentralstrahl**
Senkrecht zur Kassette, auf die Medianebene in Höhe des 4. Halswirbels.

■ **Beachte**
Medianebene von Kopf und Rumpf senkrecht zur Kassette. Der Kopf sollte durch ein Querband über die ventralen Unterkieferränder gestreckt werden.
Die Lagerung der Halswirbelsäule lässt sich durch Unterlegen eines Schaumgummikeils unter die ersten Halswirbel erleichtern.
Die Vorderextremitäten sind dabei kaudal zu fixieren.

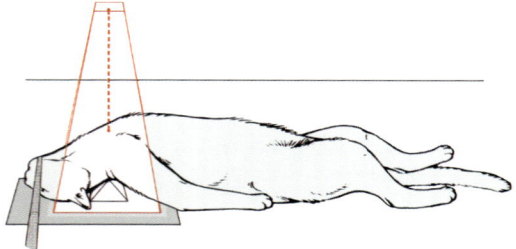

Abb. 2.3 Lagerung zur Aufnahme der Halswirbelsäule. Ventro-dorsal.

Fig. 2.3 Positioning of cervical vertebral column. Ventro-dorsal.

■ *Objective*
To image the extended, symmetric cervical vertebrae.

■ *Central ray of the primary beam*
Direct the x-ray beam perpendicular to the cassette, along the median plane centered at the level of C 4.

■ *Notice*
Align the median plane of the head and body perpendicular to the cassette, extend the head with a transverse strap over ventral borders of the mandibles.
To facilitate positioning of the vertebral column, support the more cranial cervical vertebrae with a foam rubber wedge.
The forelimbs must be fixed in a caudal direction.

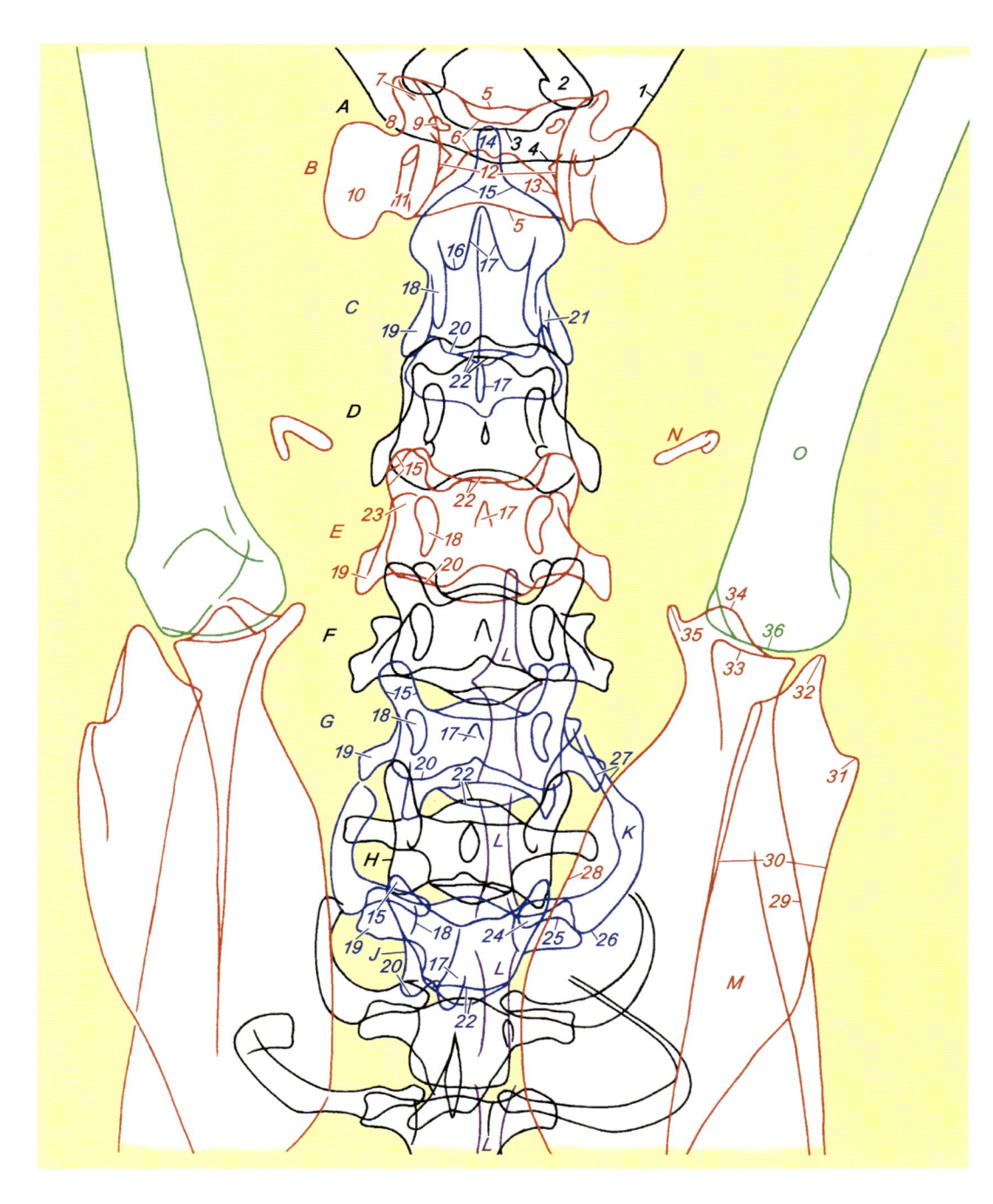

2.3 Halswirbelsäule – Cervical vertebral column ■ ventro-dorsal

A Os occipitale
1 Crista temporalis
2 Condylus occipitalis
3 Squama occipitalis
4 Crista nuchae

B Atlas
5 Arcus dorsalis
6 Arcus ventralis
7 Fovea articularis cranialis
8 Incisura alaris
9 Foramen vertebrale laterale
10 Ala atlantis
11 Foramen transversarium
12 Foramen vertebrale
13 Fovea articularis caudalis

C Axis
14 Dens
15 Processus articularis cranialis
16 Incisura vertebralis cranialis
17 Processus spinosus
18 Pediculus arcus vertebrae
19 Processus transversus
20 Processus articularis caudalis
21 Processus transversus, Tuberculum dorsale
22 Facies terminalis cranialis et caudalis

D C III

E C IV (15, 17–20, 22, siehe – see C, Axis)
23 Processus transversus, Tuberculum ventrale

F C V

G C VI (15, 17–20, 22, siehe – see C, Axis)

H C VII

J T I (15, 17–20, 22, siehe – see C, Axis)

K Os costale I
24 Caput costae
25 Collum costae
26 Tuberculum costae
27 Cartilago costae

L Sternum

M Scapula
28 Margo cranialis
29 Margo caudalis
30 Spina scapulae
31 Processus suprahamatus
32 Acromion, Processus hamatus
33 Cavitas glenoidalis
34 Tuberculum supraglenoidale
35 Processus coracoideus

N Clavicula

O Humerus
36 Caput humeri

Allgemeines zur Myelographie

Ein raumfordernder Prozess im Bereich des Wirbelkanals, der extradural (Prolapsus nuclei pulposi, Hämatom, Tumor, Metastase, Hypertrophie des Bandapparates, Abszess), intraduralextramedullär (Tumor, Zyste) oder intramedullär (Tumoren des Rückenmarkes, Hydromyelie bzw. Syringomyelie) gelegen sein kann, wird durch ein in den Subarachnoidealraum appliziertes körperwarmes, jodhaltiges (= schattengebendes) Kontrastmittel dargestellt.

Vorbereitung: Das Tier sollte nüchtern (12 Stunden keine Futteraufnahme) zur Untersuchung kommen. Vor der obligatorischen Narkose ist eine gezielte Prämedikation (entsprechend der ASA 1–5; evtl. Schmerzausschaltung) vorzunehmen und der Patient zu intubieren. Am verträglichsten ist eine Inhalationsnarkose (Isofluran/Sauerstoffgemisch), Lachgas kann bei Bedarf dazu kombiniert werden. Eine Injektionsnarkose (z.B. Propofol-Dauertropf, Dosierung: 10–15 mg/kg/h) mit Intubation und Zugabe von Sauerstoff ist ebenso gut geeignet, zur Vertiefung wird ein Opiat (z. B. Fentanyl® in einer Dosis von 0,2 mg/kg Körpermasse) kombiniert. Eine Neuroleptanalgesie wird nicht empfohlen.

Die Punktionsstellen subokzipital und lumbal werden rasiert und desinfiziert, eine Spinalkanüle mit Mandrin (z.B. 0,7 × 40 mm) vorbereitet und das Kontrastmittel angewärmt.

Kontrastmittel: Das derzeit am besten verträgliche Kontrastmittel für die Myelographie ist Jopamidol (Jopamiro®, Gerot). Diese wird als Lösung mit 200 bzw. 300 mg Jod/ml hyperosmolar zum Liquor cerebrospinalis verwendet. Es ist dünnflüssig und wasserlöslich und dissoziiert nicht. Die Neurotoxizität ist gering. Weitere mögliche Kontrastmittel sind Iohexol (Omnipaque®, Schering, bzw. Accupaque®, Nycomed) oder Iotrolan (Isovist®, Schering). Bei Tieren, die unmittelbar nach der Myelographie aufgeweckt werden, können Krämpfe auftreten, welche mit Diazepam (Valium®, Dosierung max. 1 mg/kg Körpermasse) gemildert werden.

Dosis: 0,3 bis max. 0,5 ml/kg Körpermasse; bei vermuteter Stenose im Halsbereich und subokzipitaler Punktion sollte die Dosis halbiert werden (da sonst die Kontrastmittelmenge zu beträchtlicher Druckerhöhung im subarachnoidealen Raum des Gehirns mit möglichen Konvulsionen führt).

Applikation: Das Tier wird für beide Punktionsstellen in (meist rechter) Seitenlage gelagert. Für die technisch einfachere subokzipitale Punktion wird der Kopf in der Art. atlantooccipitalis in einem etwa rechten Winkel zur Brust gebeugt, für die technisch schwierigere lumbale Punktion werden die Hinterbeine nach kranial geklappt und der Rücken gekrümmt, wodurch sich die Spatia interarcualia erweitern. Bei der subokzipitalen Punktion der Cisterna magna und/oder der lumbalen Punktion des Subarachnoidealraumes in Höhe L5/6 bzw. auch L4/5 durch das Spatium interarcuale wird (wenn nicht schon geschehen) Liquor cerebrospinalis zur chemischen und zytologischen Untersuchung gewonnen. Lumbal lässt sich trotz richtiger Kanülenlage nur selten Liquor gewinnen. Bei Verdacht auf Meningitis wird vor Ort sofort mit der Sulfosalicylsäureprobe auf Eiweiß geprüft. Als Komplikation ist bei subokzipitaler Punktion das Anstechen des dorsalen Venenplexus zu nennen. Sofortiges Zurückziehen und neuerliche Punktion mit einer frischen Kanüle können zielführend sein. Wenn bei richtigem Kanülensitz nur eine geringgradige Blutbeimengung in Form von Schlieren auftritt, kann Kontrastmittel injiziert werden.

Das körperwarme Kontrastmittel wird zügig injiziert und der Applikationsort entsprechend hochgelagert, um so ein Abfließen des spezifisch schwereren Kontrastmittels nach kaudal bzw. nach kranial zu ermöglichen.

Untersuchungstechnik: Der Fluss des Kontrastmittels ist unter Durchleuchtung gut zu verfolgen. Bei einem unveränderten, nicht unterbrochenen Subarachnoidealraum erreicht das Kontrastmittel in wenigen Minuten (3–5 Minuten) das Ende des Duralsackes lumbosakral bzw. den subokzipitalen Übergang. Nach neueren Berichten in der Literatur wird der lumbalen Applikation für thorakolumbale Prozesse der Vorzug gegeben. Die Wahrscheinlichkeit der Darstellung von Veränderungen ist aufgrund des kleineren Subarachnoidealraumes und demzufolge höheren Druckes größer als bei subokzipitaler Punktion, wo der subarachnoideale Raum des Gehirns teilweise zum Druckausgleich für das applizierte Volumen dient. Das Abfließen nach subokzipitaler Punktion allein der Schwerkraft folgend führt zu einem häufigen Stopp („Fading" aufgrund eines Rückenmarködems), der dann eine zusätzliche lumbale Punktion erfordert.

Bei einem Stopp oder einer Abweichung der Kontrastmittelsäule vom normalen Füllungsbild sind transversale, sagittale und tangentiale Aufnahmen anzufertigen, um die Art der Veränderung zu dokumentieren. Aus den teilweise typischen Füllungsbildern lässt sich in Verbindung mit dem klinischen Bild auf extradurale, intradural/extramedulläre oder intramedulläre Prozesse schließen; für einen operativen Zugang ist es wichtig, die betroffene Seite festzustellen.

Die Ausscheidung des Kontrastmittels erfolgt bereits nach 5–10 Minuten, erkennbar an der beginnenden Nierenmarkierung; die Kontrastdichte nimmt nach 20 Minuten merklich ab.

Unklare Befunde sollten frühzeitig den Schnittbildverfahren (Computertomographie bzw. Magnetresonanztomographie) zugeführt werden.

General remarks on myelography

A space-occupying lesion, situated in the vertebral canal, can be demonstrated by the introduction of an iodinated contrast medium at body temperature into the subarachnoid space. Further extradural (i.e. prolapse of the nucleus pulposus, hematoma, neoplasia, ligamentous hypertrophy, abscess), intradural- extramedullary (tumor, cyst) and intramedullary (i.e. tumor, syringo- or hydromyelia) lesions can be differentiated.

Preparation of the patient: Food should be withheld for 12 to 24 hours. Perform a selective premedication (to relieve the patient's pain), intubate the animal, and initiate general anesthesia. Inhalation anesthesia (isoflurane/oxygen, possibly in combination with nitrous oxygen) is best tolerated. Alternatively, injection anesthesia (i.e. propofol infusion at a dose of 10–15 mg/kg/h) and intubation with oxygen can be performed, in this case combined with an opiate (i.e. Fentanyl® at a dose of 0.2 mg/kg body weight) to deepen the anesthesia. Neuroleptanalgesia is not recommended. The suboccipital and lumbar site of punction are shaved and desinfected, a spinal needle and stylet (i.e. 0.7 × 40 mm) are prepared and the contrast medium is warmed.

Contrast media: Jopamidol (Jopamiro®, Gerot) is the nonionic contrast medium of choice in small animal myelography. It is applied at an iodine concentration of 200–300 mg/ml, which is hyperosmolar in comparison to the cerebrospinal liquid. It is low-viscous, water-soluble, and does not dissociate. The neurotoxicity is low. Alternate contrast media include iohexol (Omnipaque®, Schering, or Accupaque®, Nycomed) or iotrolan (Isovist®, Schering). If seizures occur during recovery from anesthesia, adminster diazepam (Valium®, intravenous at a maximum dose of 1 mg/kg body weight).

Dose: 0.3–0.5 ml/kg body weight; this dose should be reduced by one half in case of a suboccipital puncture and suspected cervical stenosis (otherwise the quantity of the contrast medium leads to increased intracranial pressure and a greater risk of seizures).

Application: Cervical myelography is performed by suboccipital puncture into the cerebellomedullary cistern with the animal in (right) lateral recumbency and with the head in a flexed position. The puncture of the lumbar subarachnoid space is more difficult than that of the cerebellomedullary cistern. It is typically performed at the level L5–6 or L4–5. The animal is positioned in lateral recumbency with the vertebral column flexed to open the interarcuate spaces.

Before the injection of contrast medium, cerebrospinal fluid is routinely removed for chemical and cytological analysis, but this is rarely possible in case of lumbar puncture. If meningitis is suspected, perform the sulfosalicylic acid test immediately in order to detect protein. A possible complication is a contamination of the sample with blood due to puncture of the venous plexus. Only an immediate withdrawal of the needle and a second puncture with a new set of needle and stylet are successful. In case of accurate positioning of the stylet and slight hemorrhagic contamination (seen as streaks), contrast injection is possible. The contrast medium should be at body temperature, and should be injected rapidly. Immediately following the injection, the injection site is elevated to aid the distribution of the contrast medium, which has a higher specific gravity than cerebrospinal fluid.

Technique: Observe the flow of the contrast medium by means of fluoroscopy. Normally, the contrast fills the subarachnoid space in about 3–5 minutes. According to new reports, the lumbar puncture is prefered, if a thoracolumbar lesion is suspected. It is thought that this is true because the volume of subarachnoid space is smaller and consequently, the subarachnoid pressure is higher. With a suboccipital puncture the greater volume of subarachnoid space compensates for the pressure gradient. Also, it is thought that the contrast column fades as it moves caudally due to spinal edema, which makes the lumbar puncture more reliable in demonstrating thoracolumbar lesions. Supplemental (lateral, ventrodorsal and oblique) projections should be made of the abnormal myelogram to document the lesion. Myelographic lesions can be grouped into the following patterns: extradural, intradural-extramedullary, and intramedullary. For surgical therapy to be successful, it is essential that the affected side is distinguished. The excretion of the contrast medium, visible by renal opacity, begins about 5–10 minutes following administration, and the opacity of the myelogram decreases significantly by 20 minutes post-injection. Questionable myelographic findings should be further evaluated by means of computed tomography or magnetic resonance imaging.

2 Wirbelsäule – Vertebral column

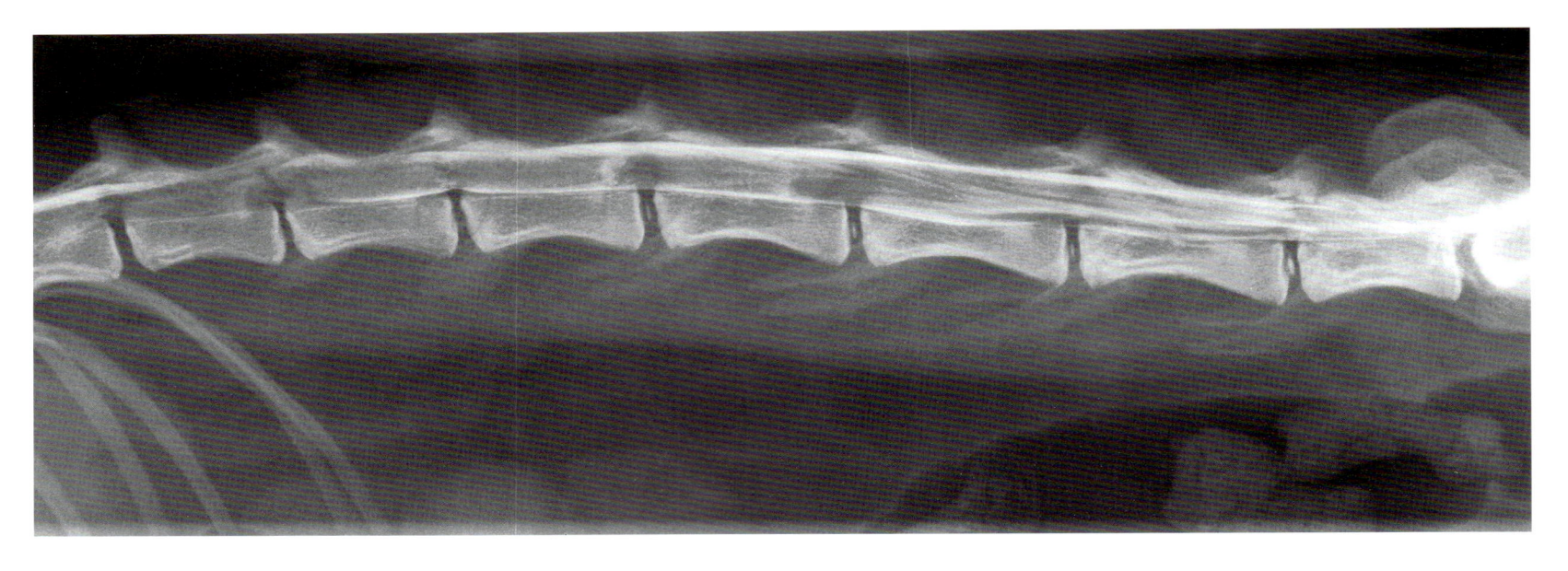

Abb. 2.4 Brust-Lenden-Wirbelsäule, latero-lateral, Myelographie
Katze
(dankenswerterweise überlassen von Frau Prof. Dr. A. TIPOLD, Hannover)

Fig. 2.4 Thoracic and lumbar vertebral column, latero-lateral, myelography
Cat
(by courtesy of Prof. Dr. A. TIPOLD, Hanover)

■ **Ziel**
Myelographische Darstellung des kontrastierten Subarachnoidealraumes am Übergang der Brust- zur Lendenwirbelsäule.

■ **Zentralstrahl**
Senkrecht zur Kassette, in Höhe des 3.–4. Lendenwirbels.

■ **Beachte**
Streckung der Schultergliedmaßen nach vorn und der Beckengliedmaßen nach hinten.

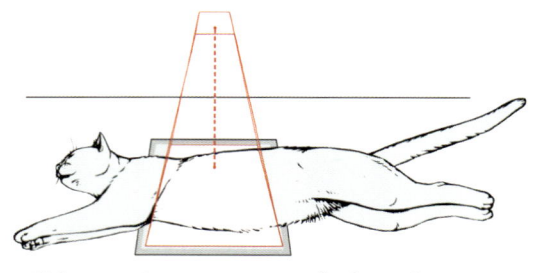

Abb. 2.4 Lagerung zur Aufnahme der Brust-Lenden-Wirbelsäule. Latero-lateral.

Fig. 2.4 Positioning of the thoracic and lumbar vertebral column. Latero-lateral.

■ *Objective*
To image by myelography the subarachnoidal space in the thoracic and lumbar regions.

■ *Central ray of the primary beam*
Direct the x-ray beam perpendicular to the cassette, centered in the middle of L3–4.

■ *Notice*
Stretch the thoracic limbs cranially and the pelvic limbs caudally.

2.4 Myelographie, Brust-Lenden-Wirbelsäule – Myelography, Thoracic and lumbar vertebral column ■ latero-lateral

A	L1	1	Cavum subarachnoideale, dorsal, mit Kontrastmittel – *with contrast medium*	a	Innere Lendenmuskeln – *inner lumbar muscles*
B	L2	2	Cavum subarachnoideale, ventral, mit Kontrastmittel – *with contrast medium*	b	Ren dexter
C	L7			c	Ren sinister
D	Ala ossi ilii, D´ plattenfern – *next to the tube*	3	Nucleus pulposus in Protrusion (L1 – L2)	d	Colon descendens
E	Os costale XIII	4	Radices nervi spinales, mit Kontrastmittel – *with contrast medium*		

2 Wirbelsäule – Vertebral column

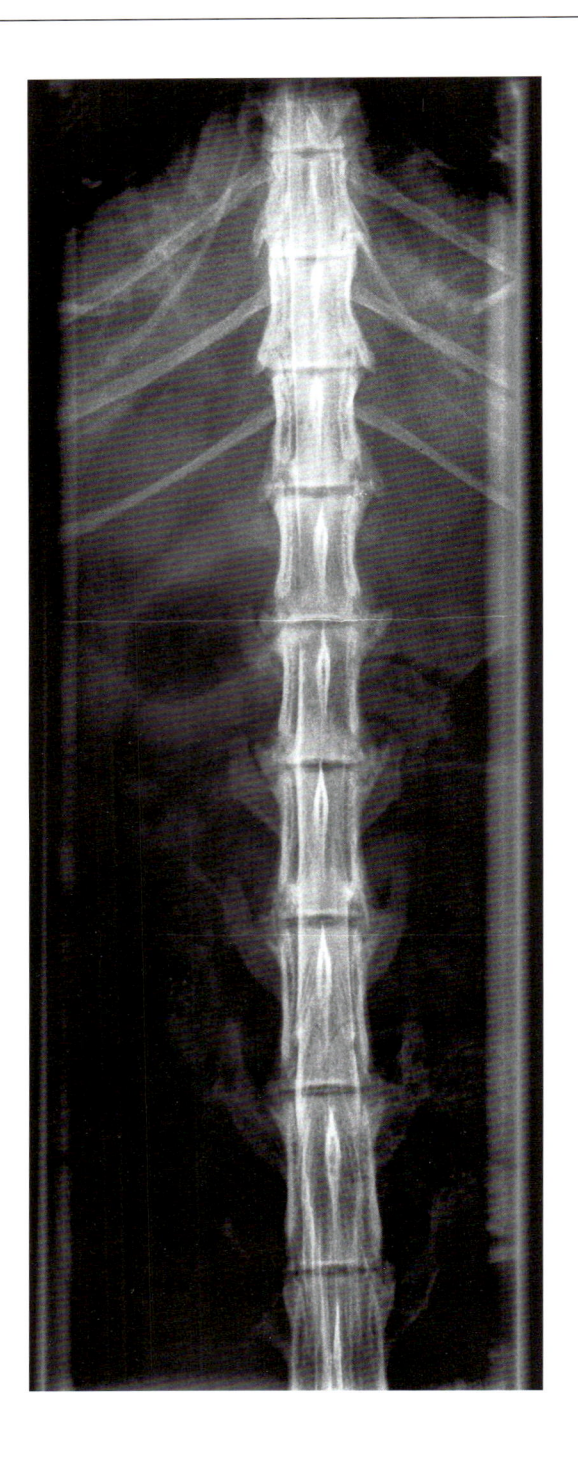

Abb. 2.5 Brust-Lenden-Wirbelsäule, ventro-dorsal, Myelographie
Katze
(dankenswerterweise überlassen von Frau Prof. Dr. A. TIPOLD, Hannover)

Fig. 2.5 Thoracic and lumbar vertebral column, ventro-dorsal, myelography
Cat
(by courtesy of Prof. Dr. A. TIPOLD, Hanover)

■ **Ziel**
Myelographische Darstellung des kontrastierten Subarachnoidealraumes am Übergang der Brust- zur Lendenwirbelsäule.

■ **Zentralstrahl**
Senkrecht zur Kassette, auf die Medianebene, in Höhe des 3. Lendenwirbels.

■ **Beachte**
Streckung der Schultergliedmaßen nach vorn und der Beckengliedmaßen nach hinten.

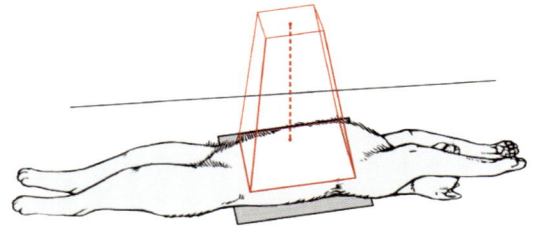

Abb. 2.5 Lagerung zur Aufnahme der Brust-Lenden-Wirbelsäule. Ventro-dorsal.

Fig. 2.5 Positioning of thoracic and vertebral column. Ventro-dorsal.

■ *Objective*
To image by myelography the subarachnoidal space in the thoracic and lumbar regions.

■ *Central ray of the primary beam*
Direct the x-ray beam perpendicular to the cassette, along the median plane, centered at the level of L3.

■ *Notice*
Stretch the thoracic limbs cranially and the pelvic limbs caudally.

2.5 Myelographie, Brust-Lenden-Wirbelsäule – Myelography, Thoracic and lumbar vertebral column ■ ventro-dorsal

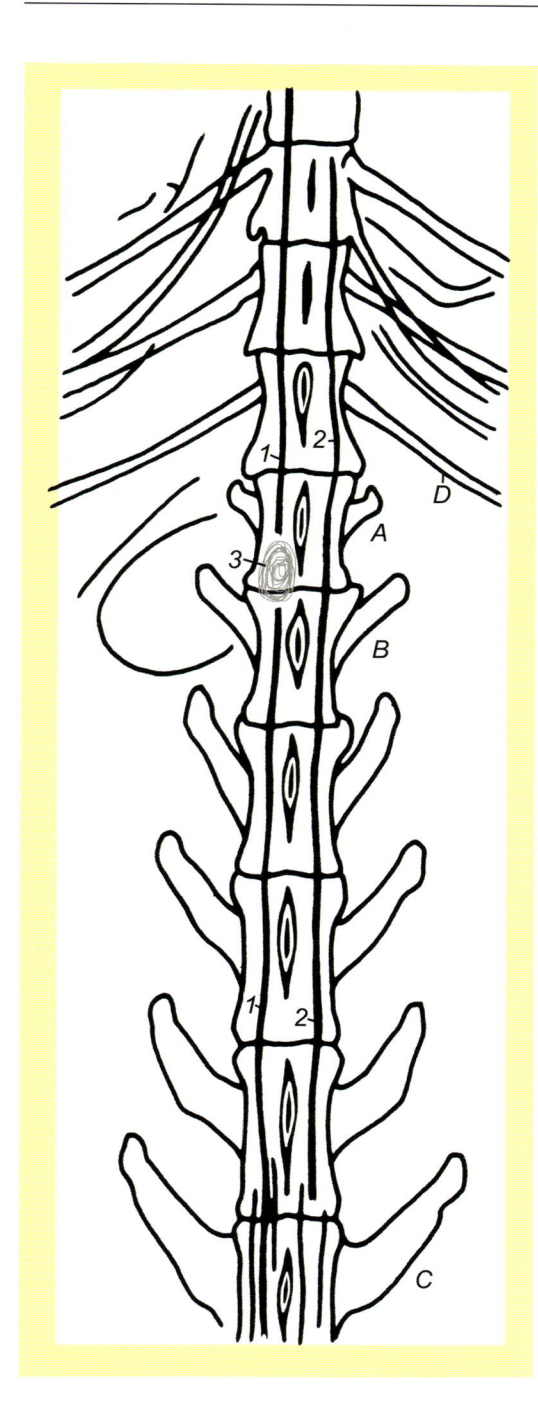

A	L1
B	L2
C	L7
D	Os costale XIII
1	Cavum subarachnoideale, links, mit Kontrastmittel – *left with contrast medium*
2	Cavum subarachnoideale, rechts, mit Kontrastmittel – *right with contrast medium*
3	Nucleus pulposus in Protrusion (L1–L2)

3 Schultergliedmaße – Thoracic limb

A Humerus
1. Collum humeri
2. Tuberculum majus
3. Caput humeri

B Scapula, B´ plattenfern – *next to the tube*
4. Cavitas glenoidalis
5. Acromion, Processus hamatus
6. Tuberculum supraglenoidale
7. Processus coracoideus
8. Processus suprahamatus
9. Spina scapulae, Basis, 9´ plattenfern – *next to the tube*
10. Spina scapulae, Rand – *border*
11. Margo caudalis
12. Angulus caudalis
13. Margo dorsalis
14. Angulus cranialis
15. Margo cranialis

C Clavicula, C´ plattenfern – *next to the tube*

D C V

E T I

F Os costale I, F´ plattenfern – *next to the tube*

G Manubrium sterni

H Trachea

Abb. 3.1 Rechtes Schultergelenk, medio-lateral,
Katze
(Ausschnitt aus 13 × 18 cm)

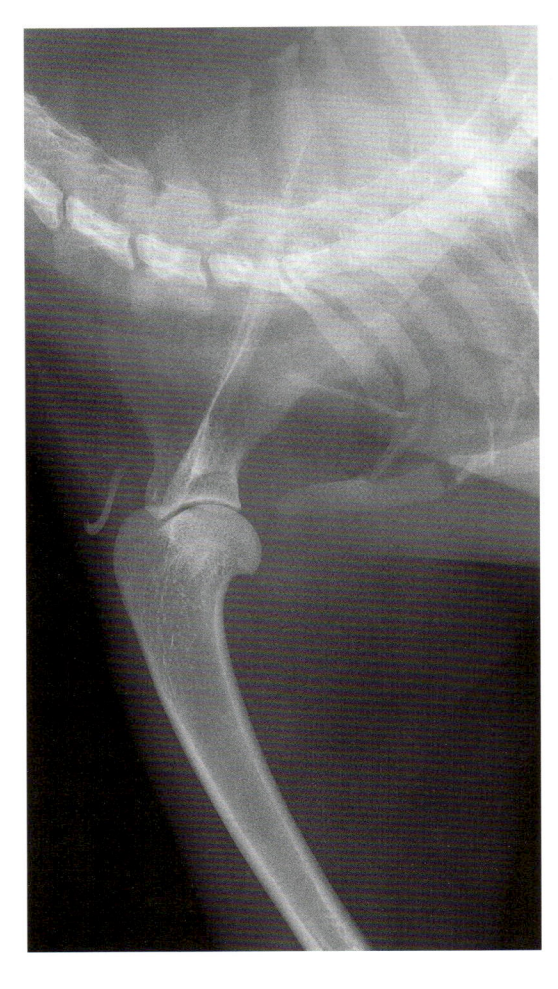

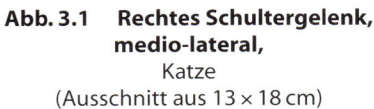

Fig. 3.1 Right shoulder joint, medio-lateral,
Cat
(section of 13 × 18 cm)

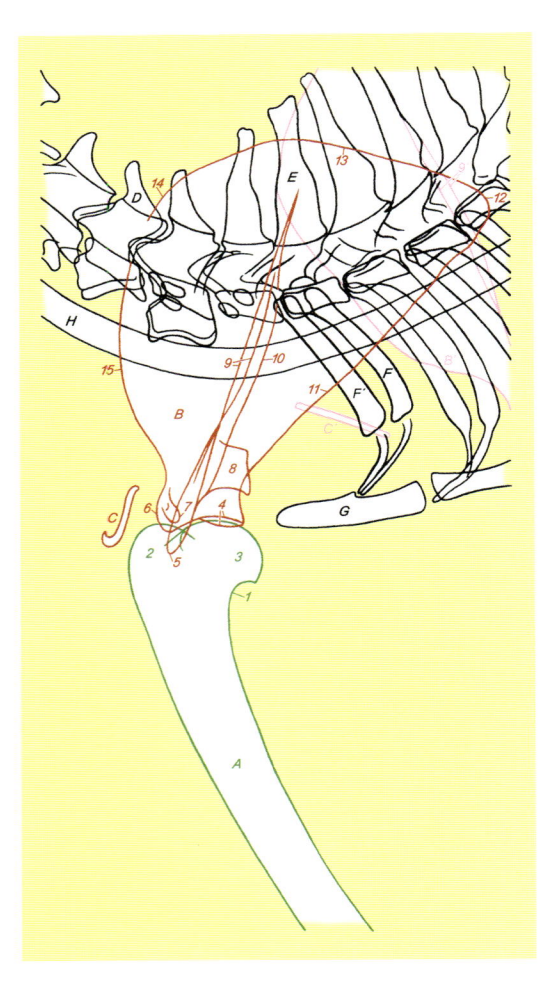

■ Ziel
Darstellung eines Schultergelenks, ohne Überlagerung durch den Hals oder Brustkorb.

■ Zentralstrahl
Senkrecht zur Kassette, dicht kaudal des Tuberculum majus humeri.

■ Beachte
Unten liegende (zu untersuchende) Gliedmaße nach vorn strecken, während die oben liegende Gliedmaße nach hinten verlagert wird; Kopf und Hals nach dorsal strecken.

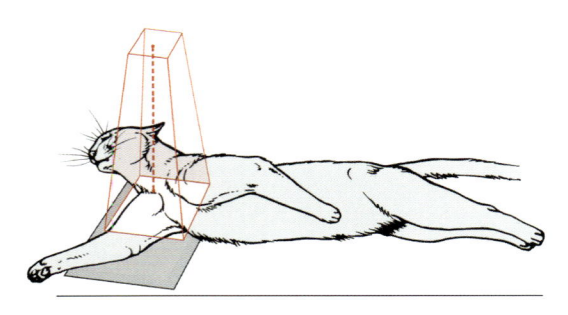

Abb 3.1 Lagerung zur Aufnahme des Schultergelenks. Medio-lateral.

Fig. 3.1 Positioning of shoulder joint. Medio-lateral.

■ *Objective*
To image the shoulder joint without superimposition of the neck or thorax.

■ *Central ray of the primary beam*
Direct the x-ray beam perpendicular to the cassette, centered slightly caudal to the greater tubercle of the humerus.

■ *Notice*
The patient lies on the side of interest, stretch the dependent limb cranially and the nondependent limb caudally; extend head and neck dorsally.

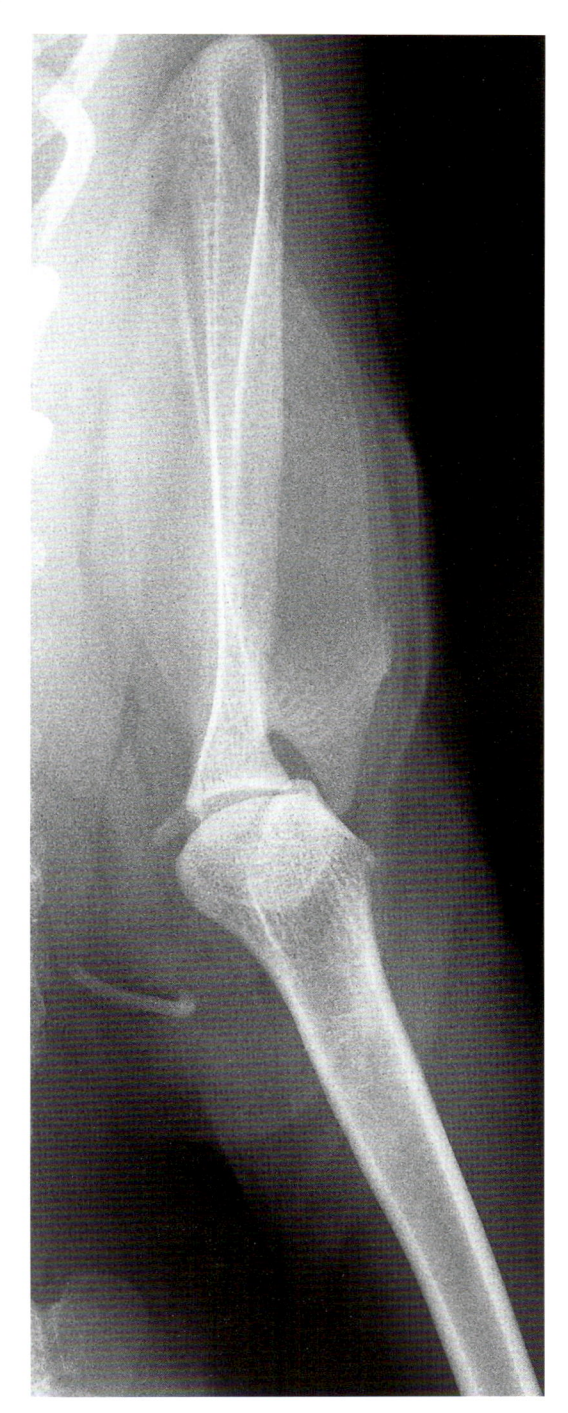

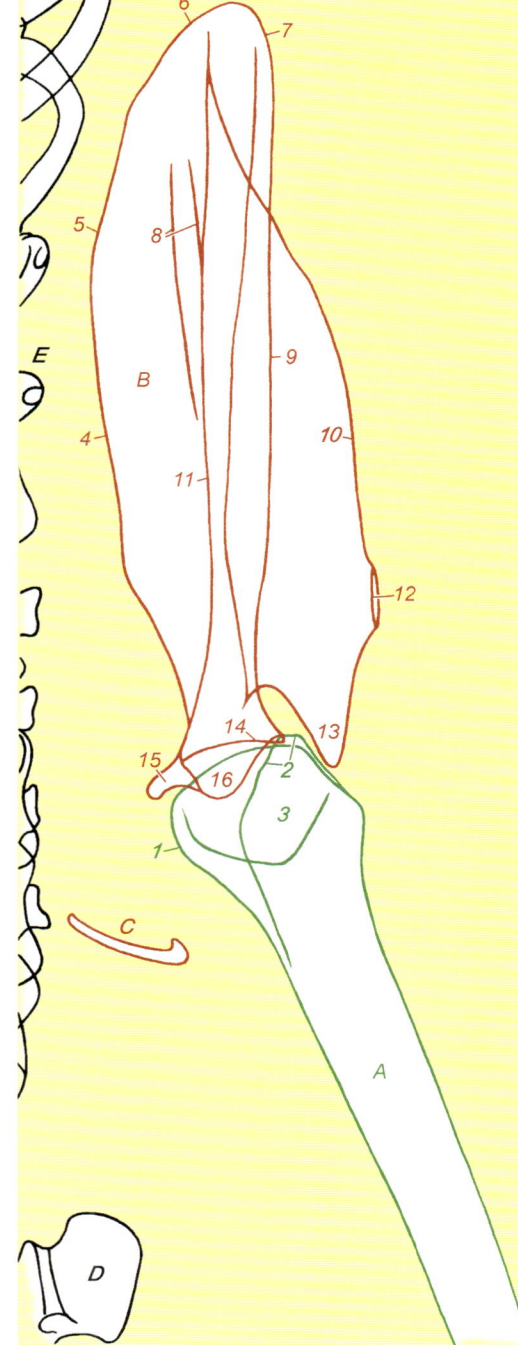

3.2 Linkes Schultergelenk – Left shoulder joint ■ kaudo-kranial – caudo-cranial

A Humerus
1 Tuberculum minus
2 Tuberculum majus
3 Caput humeri

B Scapula
4 Margo cranialis
5 Angulus cranialis
6 Margo dorsalis
7 Angulus caudalis
8 Muskelleisten – *crests of muscle attachments*
9 Margo caudalis scapulae
10 Spina scapulae, Rand – *border*
11 Spina scapulae, Basis
12 Processus suprahamatus
13 Acromion, Processus hamatus
14 Cavitas glenoidalis
15 Processus coracoideus
16 Tuberculum supraglenoidale

C Clavicula

D Atlas

E Os costale II

Abb. 3.2 Linkes Schultergelenk, kaudo-kranial,
Katze
(Ausschnitt aus 13 × 18 cm)

Fig. 3.2 Left shoulder joint, caudo-cranial,
Cat
(section of 13 × 18 cm)

■ **Ziel**
Darstellung der Gelenkflächen des Schultergelenks.

■ **Zentralstrahl**
Senkrecht zur Kassette, auf die Mitte der kaudalen Gliedmaßenfläche in die Beuge des Schultergelenks.

■ **Beachte**
Beide Schultergliedmaßen seitlich am Kopf fixieren, so dass die Ellbogenhöcker nach oben zeigen.

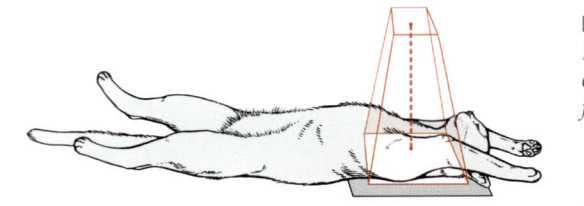

Abb. 3.2 Lagerung zur Aufnahme des Schultergelenks. Kaudo-kranial.

Fig. 3.2 Positioning of shoulder joint. Caudo-cranial.

■ *Objective*
To image the articular surfaces of the shoulder joint.

■ *Central ray of the primary beam*
Direct the x-ray beam perpendicular to the cassette, centered on the caudal surface of the limb, at the flexion side of the shoulder joint.

■ *Notice*
Fix both thoracic limbs to the lateral aspect of the head, so that both tuber olecrani show upwards.

43

3 Schultergliedmaße – Thoracic limb

A Scapula
1 Spina scapulae
2 Processus suprahamatus
3 Acromion, Processus hamatus
4 Collum scapulae
5 Cavitas glenoidalis
6 Tuberculum supraglenoidale et Processus coracoideus

B Clavicula

C Humerus
7 Caput humeri
8 Tuberculum minus
9 Tuberculum majus
10 Tuberositas deltoidea
11 Corpus humeri
12 Crista supracondylaris lateralis
13 Fossa radialis
14 Capitulum humeri, kranialer Rand – *cranial border*
15 Capitulum humeri
16 Trochlea humeri, ventraler Rand – *ventral border*
17 Epicondylus medialis
18 Epicondylus lateralis
19 Fossa olecrani

D Ulna
20 Tuber olecrani
21 Olecranon
22 Processus anconaeus
23 Incisura trochlearis
24 Processus coronoideus lateralis
25 Processus coronoideus medialis

E Radius
26 Caput radii
27 Collum radii
28 Tuberositas radii

Abb. 3.3 Linker Oberarm, medio-lateral,
Katze
(Ausschnitt aus 13 × 18 cm)

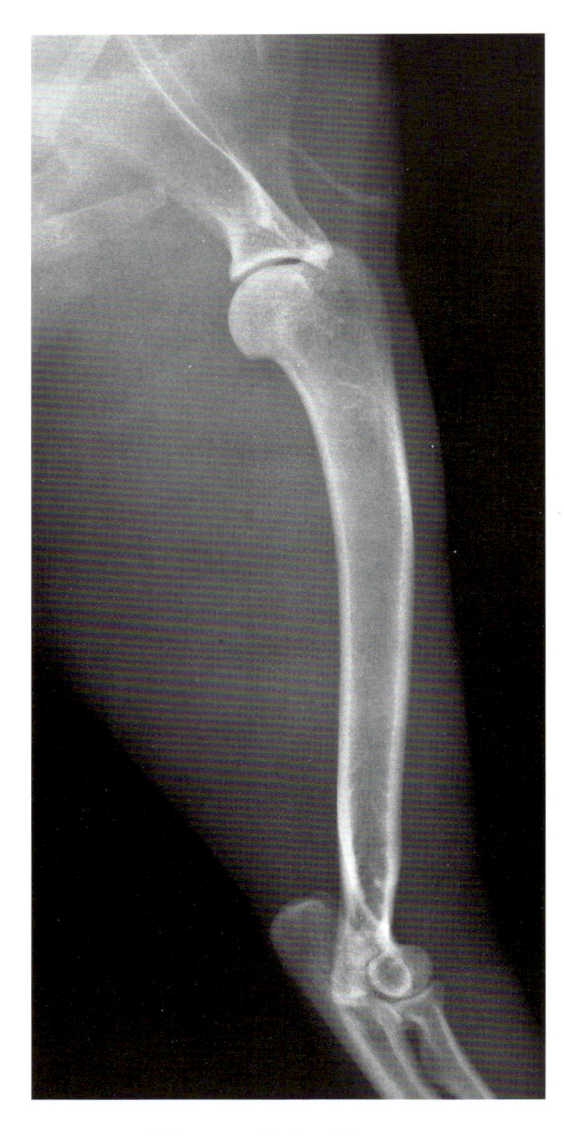

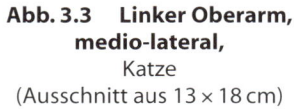

Fig. 3.3 Left arm, medio-lateral,
Cat
(section of 13 × 18 cm)

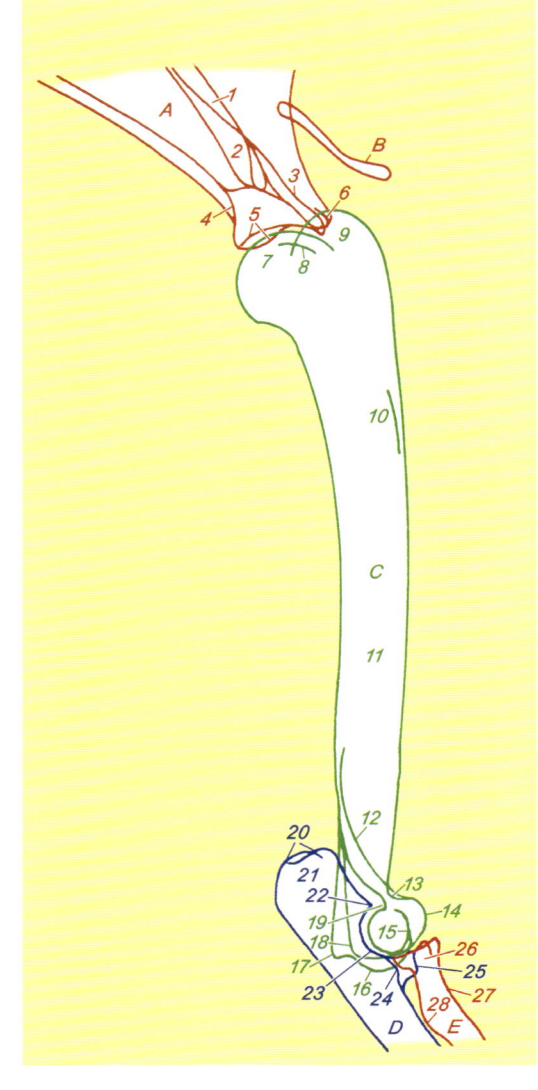

■ **Ziel**
Darstellung des Oberarms mit Schulter- und Ellbogengelenk, ohne Überlagerung durch den Hals oder Brustkorb.

■ **Zentralstrahl**
Senkrecht zur Kassette, medial in Höhe der Schaftmitte des Humerus.

■ **Beachte**
Unten liegende (zu untersuchende) Gliedmaße nach vorn strecken, während die oben liegende Gliedmaße nach hinten verlagert wird; Kopf und Hals nach dorsal strecken.
Schulter- und Ellbogengelenk müssen mit abgebildet sein.

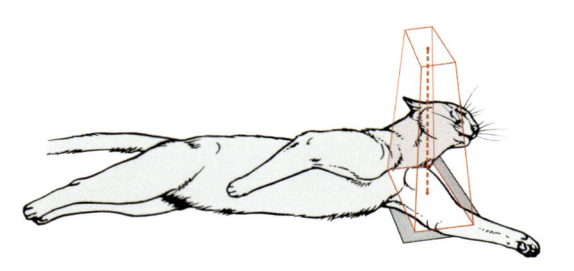

Abb. 3.3 Lagerung zur Aufnahme des Oberarms. Medio-lateral.

Fig. 3.3 Positioning of the arm. Medio-lateral.

■ *Objective*
To image the arm including shoulder and elbow joints, without superimposition of the neck or thorax.

■ *Central ray of the primary beam*
Direct the x-ray beam perpendicular to the cassette, centered in the middle of the humerus.

■ *Notice*
The patient lies on the side of interest, stretch the dependent limb cranially and the nondependent limb caudally; extend head and neck dorsally.
The shoulder and elbow joints should be imaged.

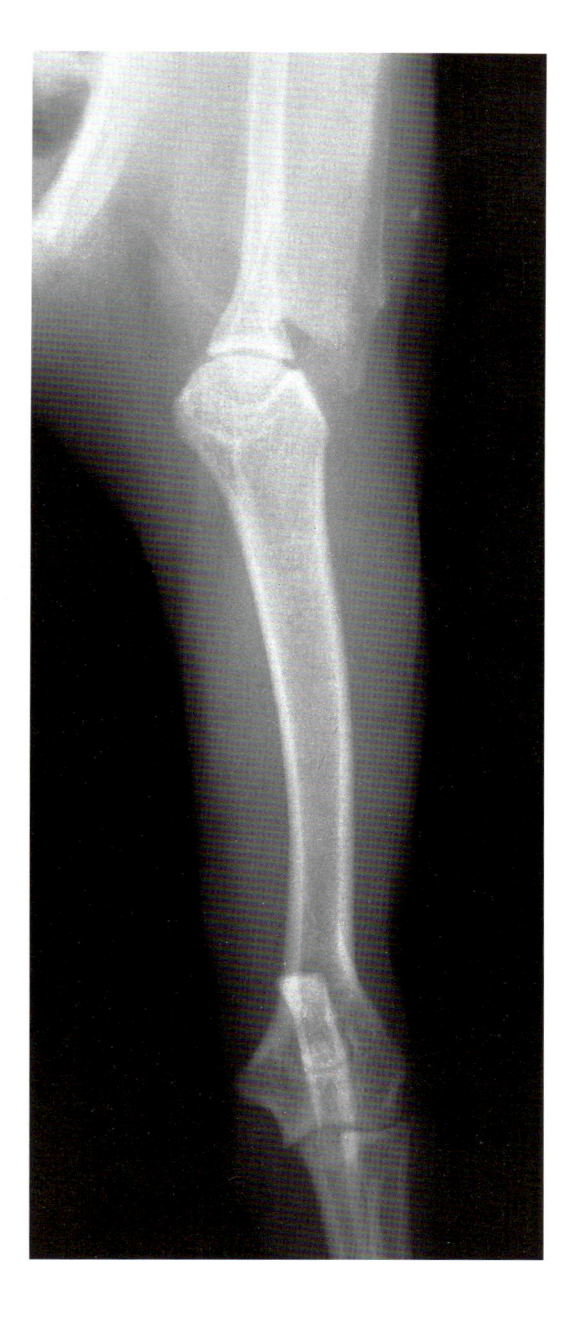

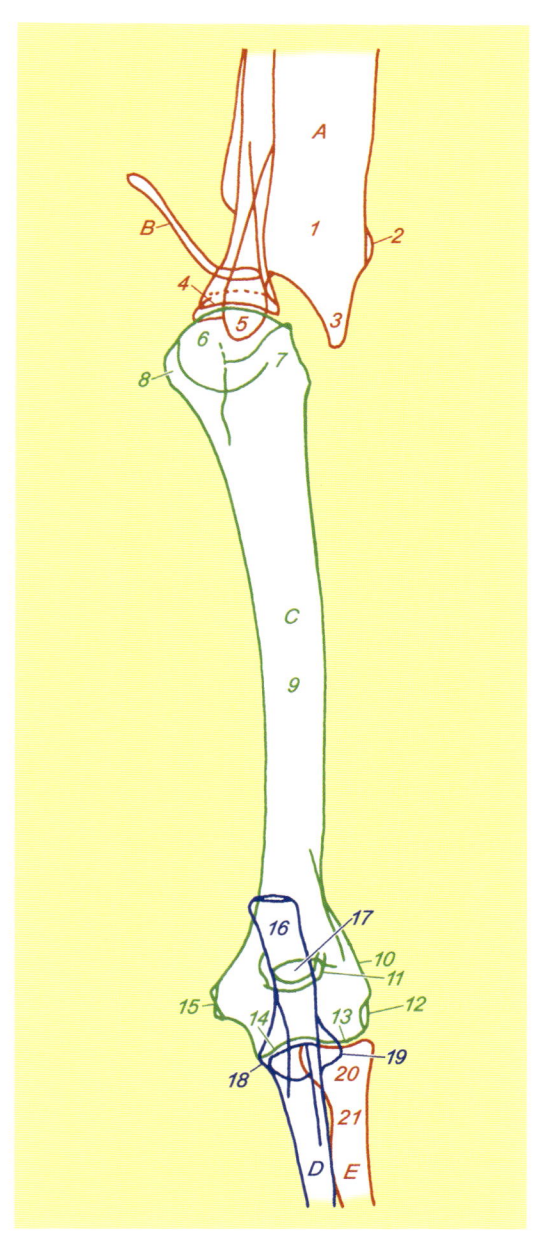

3.4 Linker Oberarm – Left arm ■ kaudo-kranial – caudo-cranial

A **Scapula**
1 Spina scapulae
2 Processus suprahamatus
3 Acromion, Processus hamatus
4 Cavitas glenoidalis
5 Tuberculum supraglenoidale

B **Clavicula**

C **Humerus**
6 Caput humeri
7 Tuberculum majus
8 Tuberculum minus
9 Corpus humeri
10 Epicondylus lateralis
11 Fossa olecrani
12 Bandgrube – *depression for ligamentous attachment*
13 Capitulum humeri
14 Trochlea humeri
15 Epicondylus medialis

D **Ulna**
16 Olecranon
17 Processus anconaeus
18 Processus coronoideus medialis
19 Processus coronoideus lateralis

E **Radius**
20 Caput radii
21 Collum radii

Abb. 3.4 Linker Oberarm, kaudo-kranial,
Katze
(Ausschnitt aus 18 x 24 cm)

Fig. 3.4 Left arm, caudo-cranial,
Cat
(section of 18 x 24 cm)

■ **Ziel**
Darstellung des Oberarms mit Schulter- und Ellbogengelenk.

■ **Zentralstrahl**
Senkrecht zur Kassette, kranial in Höhe der kaudalen Schaftmitte.

■ **Beachte**
Beide Gliedmaßen nach vorn strecken; Kopf und Hals möglichst weit nach dorsal strecken; nicht verkanten!

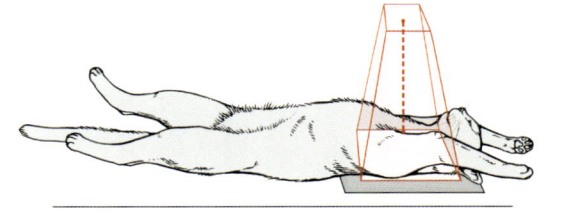

Abb. 3.4 Lagerung zur Aufnahme des Oberarms. Kaudo-kranial.

Fig. 3.4 Positioning of the arm. Caudo-cranial.

■ *Objective*
To image the arm including the shoulder and elbow joints.

■ *Central ray of the primary beam*
Direct the x-ray beam perpendicular to the cassette, centered in the middle of the caudal surface of the limb.

■ *Notice*
Stretch both limbs cranially; extend head and neck completely; do not tilt!

3 Schultergliedmaße – Thoracic limb

A Humerus
1	Foramen supracondylare
2	Fossa olecrani
3	Epicondylus lateralis
4	Epicondylus medialis
5	Capitulum humeri
6	Trochlea humeri

B Ulna
7	Tuber olecrani, kaudaler Höcker – *caudal tubercle*
8	Tuber olecrani, kraniolateraler Höcker – *craniolateral tubercle*
9	Tuber olecrani, kraniomedialer Höcker – *craniomedial tubercle*
10	Processus anconaeus
11	Incisura trochlearis
12	Processus coronoideus lateralis
13	Processus coronoideus medialis

C Radius
14	Tuberositas radii
15	Spatium interosseum antebrachii

Abb. 3.5 Rechtes Ellbogengelenk, medio-lateral,
Katze
(Ausschnitt aus 13 × 18 cm)

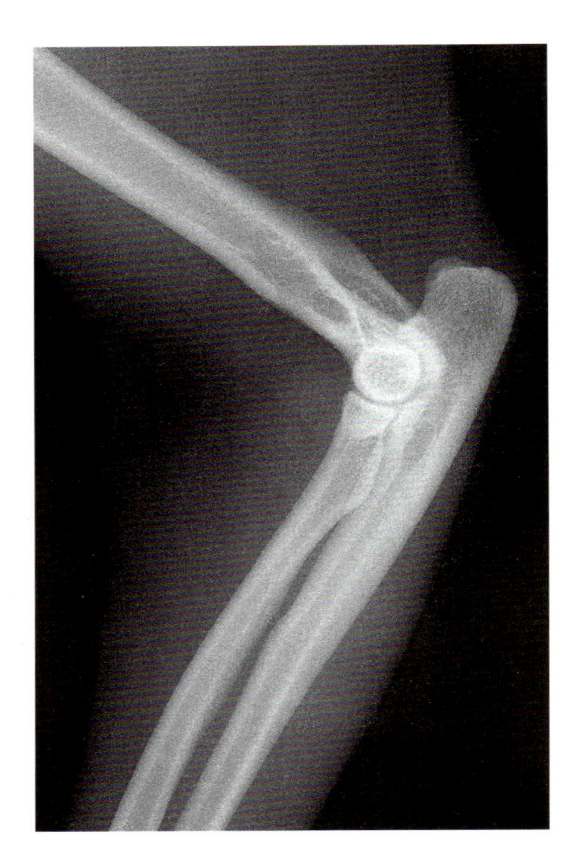

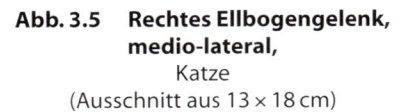

Fig. 3.5 Right elbow joint, medio-lateral,
Cat
(section of 13 × 18 cm)

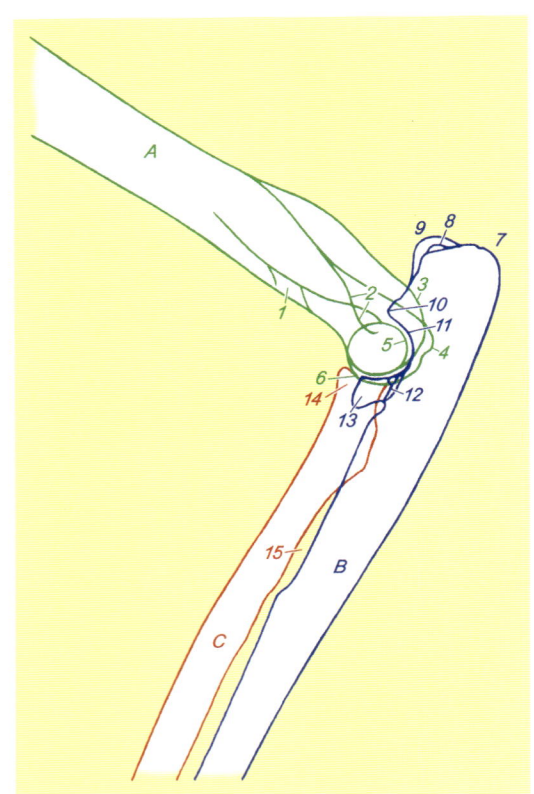

■ **Ziel**
Darstellung des Ellbogengelenks, speziell des Condylus humeri, des Olekranon, des Caput radii und des Processus coronoideus medialis.

■ **Zentralstrahl**
Senkrecht zur Kassette, medial in Höhe des palpierbaren Epicondylus medialis humeri.

■ **Beachte**
Unten liegende (zu untersuchende) Gliedmaße etwas nach vorn strecken, während die oben liegende Gliedmaße nach hinten verlagert wird; Kopf und Hals nach dorsal strecken.

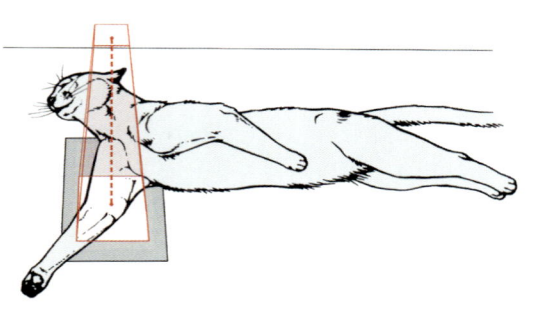

Abb. 3.5 Lagerung zur Aufnahme des Ellbogengelenks. Medio-lateral.

Fig. 3.5 Positioning of the elbow joint. Medio-lateral.

■ *Objective*
To image the elbow joint, especially the humeral condyle, the olecranon, the radial head, and the medial coronoid process of the ulna.

■ *Central ray of the primary beam*
Direct the x-ray beam perpendicular to the cassette, centered on the palpable medial epicondyle of the humerus.

■ *Notice*
The patient lies on the side of interest, stretch the dependent limb cranially and the nondependent limb caudally to the dependent stifle; extend the head and neck dorsally.

3.6 Rechtes Ellbogengelenk – Right elbow joint ■ kranio-kaudal – cranio-caudal

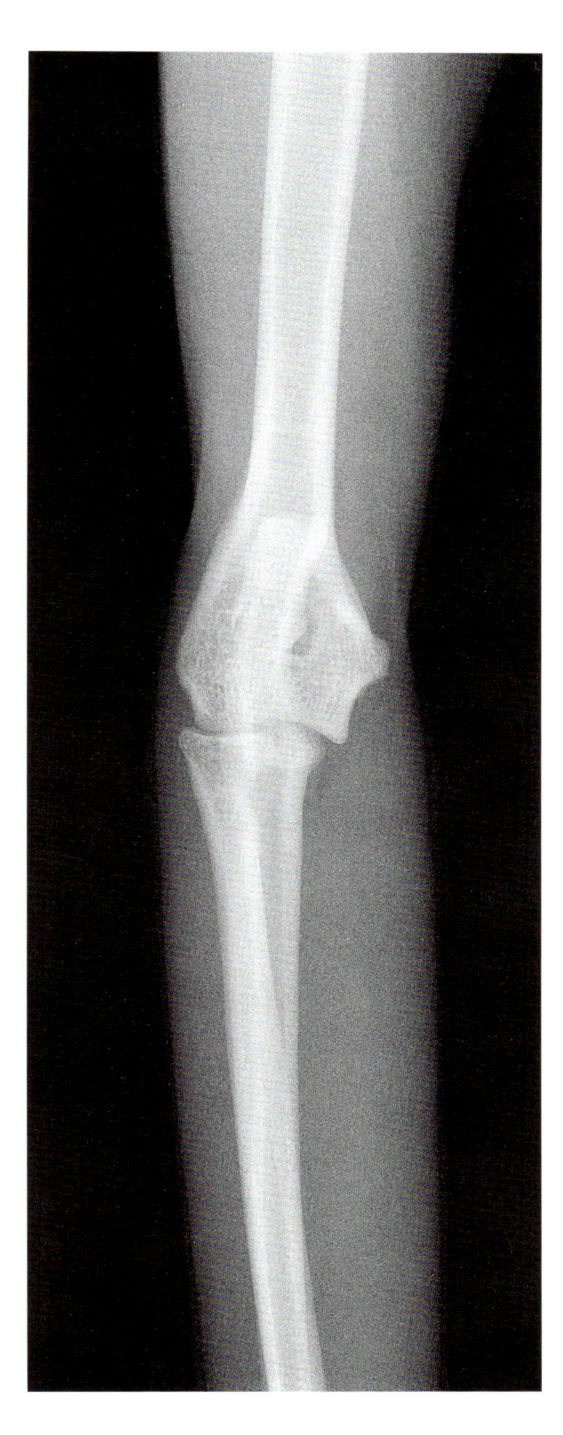

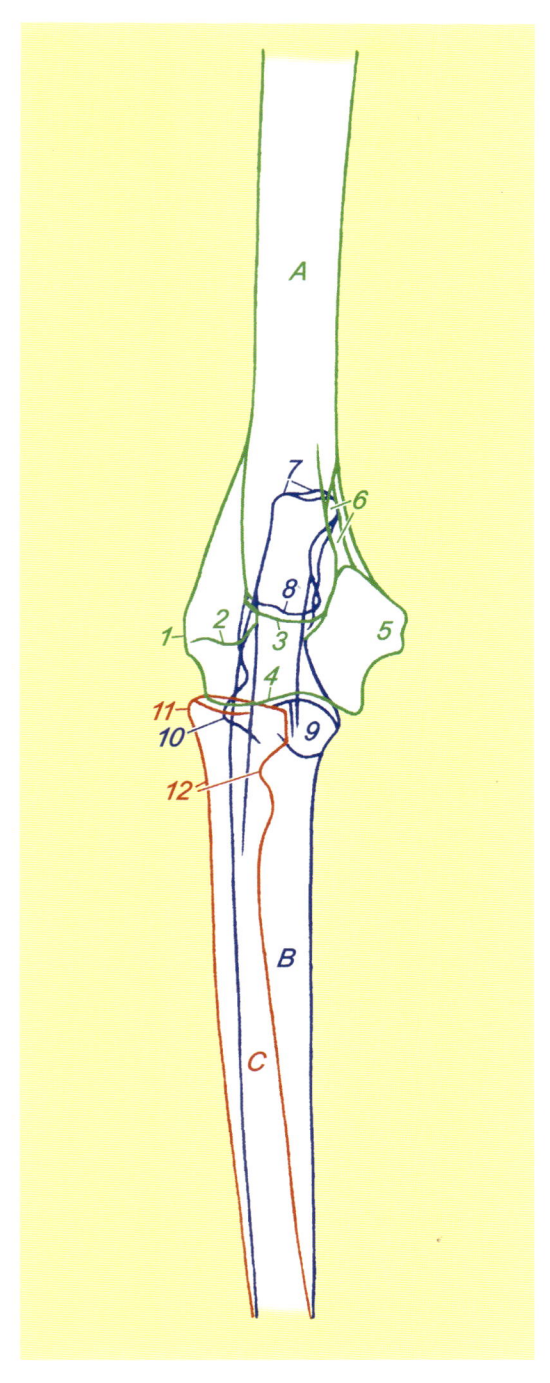

Abb. 3.6 Rechtes Ellbogengelenk, kranio-kaudal,
Katze
(Ausschnitt aus 13 × 18 cm)

Fig. 3.6 Right elbow joint, cranio-caudal,
Cat
(section of 13 × 18 cm)

A Humerus
1 Epicondylus lateralis
2 Capitulum humeri, kranialer Rand der Gelenkfläche – *cranial border of articular surface*
3 Fossa olecrani
4 Trochlea humeri
5 Epicondylus medialis
6 Foramen supracondylare

B Ulna
7 Tuber olecrani
8 Processus anconeus
9 Processus coronoideus medialis
10 Processus coronoideus lateralis

C Radius
11 Caput radii
12 Collum radii

■ **Ziel**
Darstellung des Ellbogengelenks, speziell des horizontalen Gelenkspaltes und des Condylus humeri (Trochlea und Capitulum).

■ **Zentralstrahl**
Senkrecht zur Kassette, kranial des palpierbaren Gelenkspalts.

■ **Beachte**
Beide Gliedmaßen nach vorn strecken; Kopf und Hals möglichst weit nach dorsal strecken; nicht verkanten!

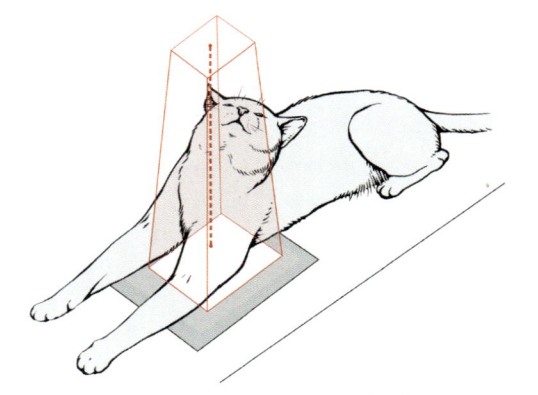

Abb. 3.6 Lagerung zur Aufnahme des Ellbogengelenks. Kranio-kaudal.

Fig. 3.6 Positioning of the elbow joint. Cranio-caudal.

■ *Objective*
To image the elbow joint, especially of the horizontal joint space and the humeral condyle (trochlea and capitulum).

■ *Central ray of the primary beam*
Direct the x-ray beam perpendicular to the cassette, centered at the level of the joint space.

■ *Notice*
Stretch both limbs cranially; extend the head and neck dorsally; do not tilt!

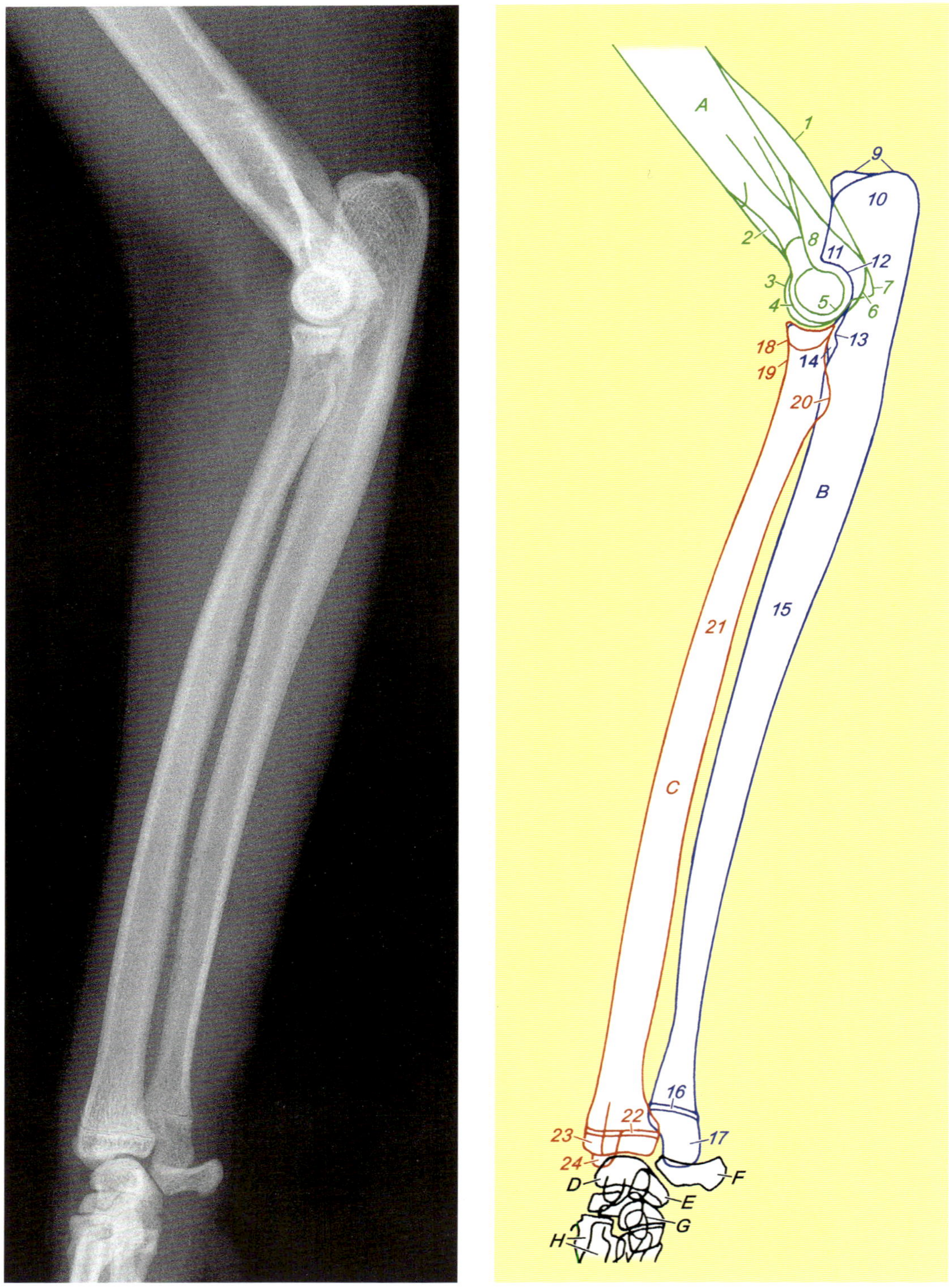

3 Schultergliedmaße – Thoracic limb

A Humerus
1. Crista supracondylaris lateralis
2. Foramen supracondylare
3. Trochlea humeri, medialer Rand – *medial border*
4. Capitulum, lateraler Rand – *lateral border*
5. Trochlea humeri, Führungsrinne – *groove*
6. Epicondylus lateralis
7. Epicondylus medialis
8. Fossa olecrani

B Ulna
9. Tuber olecrani
10. Olecranon
11. Processus anconaeus
12. Incisura trochlearis
13. Processus coronoideus lateralis
14. Processus coronoideus medialis
15. Corpus ulnae
16. Epiphysenfugenknorpel – *cartilage of the epiphyseal plate*
17. Caput ulnae et Processus styloideus

C Radius
18. Caput radii
19. Collum radii
20. Tuberositas radii
21. Corpus radii
22. distaler Epiphysenfugenknorpel – *cartilage of the distal epiphyseal plate*
23. Epiphysis distalis, Trochlea radii
24. Processus styloideus radii

D Os carpi intermedioradiale

E Os carpi ulnare

F Os carpi accessorium

G Ossa carpalia I–IV, mit Überlagerungen – *in superposition*

H Ossa metacarpalia

Abb. 3.7 Rechter Unterarm, medio-lateral,
Katze
(Ausschnitt aus 13 × 18 cm)

Fig. 3.7 Right forearm, medio-lateral,
Cat
(section of 13 × 18 cm)

■ **Ziel**
Darstellung des Unterarms mit Ellbogen- und Karpalgelenk.

■ **Zentralstrahl**
Senkrecht zur Kassette, medial in Höhe der Schaftmitte des Radius.

■ **Beachte**
Unten liegende (zu untersuchende) Gliedmaße etwas nach vorn strecken, während die oben liegende Gliedmaße nach hinten verlagert wird; Kopf und Hals nach dorsal strecken.

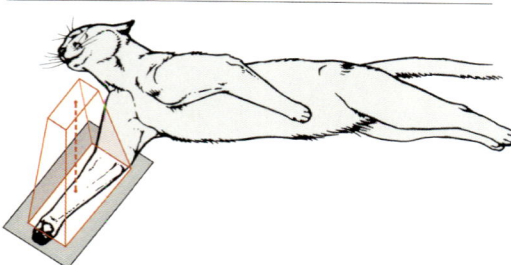

Abb. 3.7 Lagerung zur Aufnahme des Unterarms. Medio-lateral.

Fig. 3.7 Positioning of the forearm. Medio-lateral.

■ *Objective*
To image the forearm, including the elbow and carpal joints.

■ *Central ray of the primary beam*
Direct the x-ray beam perpendicular to the cassette, centered in the middle of the radius.

■ *Notice*
The patient lies on the side of interest, stretch the dependent limb cranially and the nondependent limb caudally to the dependent stifle; extend the head and neck dorsally.

3.8 Rechter Unterarm – Right forearm ■ kranio-kaudal – cranio-caudal

A Humerus
1. Foramen supracondylare
2. Fossa olecrani
3. Epicondylus medialis
4. Trochlea humeri
5. Capitulum humeri
6. Epicondylus lateralis

B Ulna
7. Tuber olecrani
8. Processus anconaeus
9. Incisura trochlearis
10. Processus coronoideus lateralis
11. Processus coronoideus medialis
12. Corpus ulnae
13. Epiphysenfugenknorpel – cartilage of the epiphyseal plate
14. Caput ulnae et Processus styloideus

C Radius
15. Caput radii
16. Collum radii
17. Corpus radii
18. distaler Epiphysenfugenknorpel – cartilage of the distal epiphyseal plate
19. Trochlea radii
20. Processus styloideus radii

D Os carpi intermedioradiale

E Os carpi ulnare

F Os carpi accessorium

G Ossa carpalia I–IV

H Ossa metacarpalia I–V

J Os sesamoideum m. abductoris pollicis longi

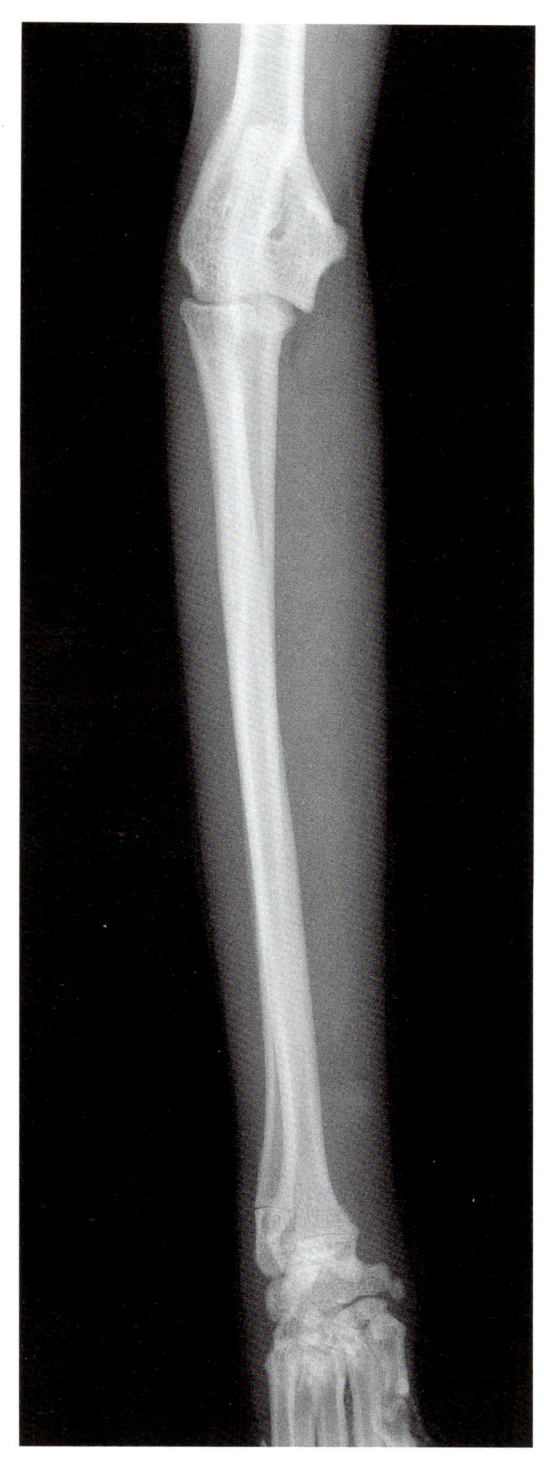

Abb. 3.8 Rechter Unterarm, kranio-kaudal,
Katze
(Ausschnitt aus 13 × 18 cm)

Fig. 3.8 Right forearm, cranio-caudal,
Cat
(section of 13 × 18 cm)

■ **Ziel**
Darstellung des Unterarms mit Ellbogen- und Karpalgelenk.

■ **Zentralstrahl**
Senkrecht zur Kassette, kranial in Höhe Schaftmitte des Radius.

■ **Beachte**
Beide Gliedmaßen nach vorn strecken. Kopf und Hals möglichst weit nach dorsal strecken; nur der Kaudalrand des Olekranon berührt die Kassette; nicht verkanten!

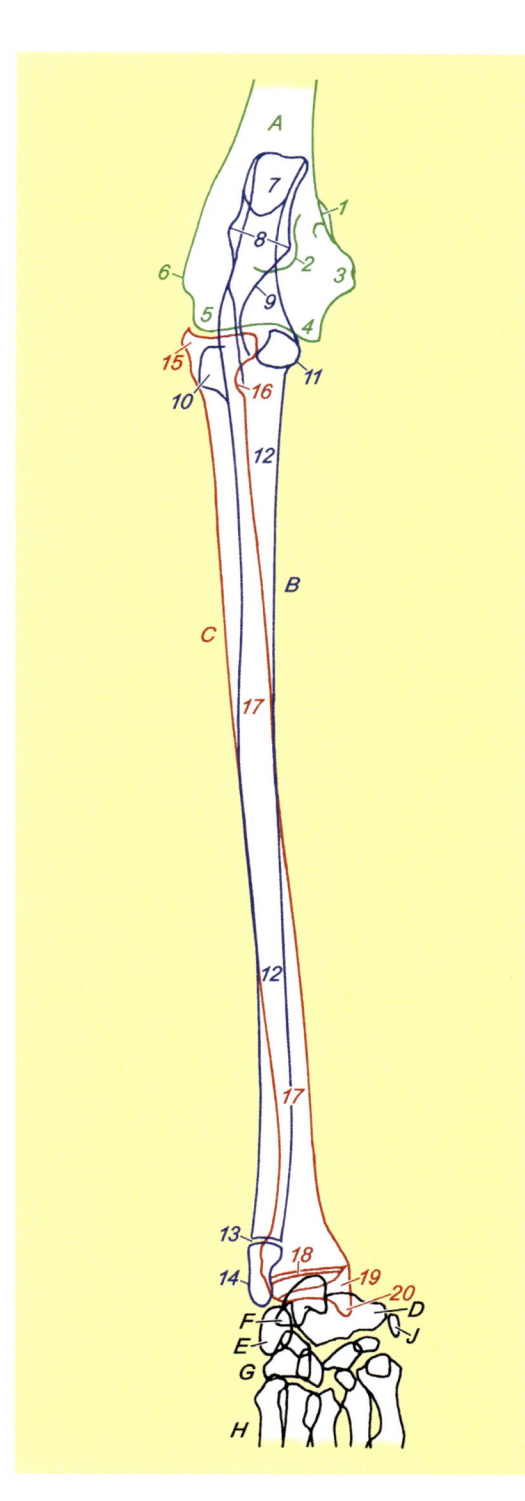

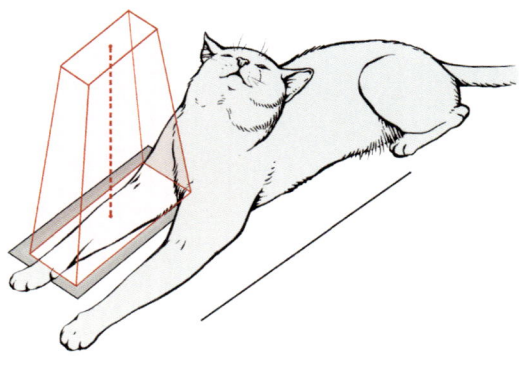

Abb. 3.8 Lagerung zur Aufnahme des Unterarms. Kranio-kaudal.

Fig. 3.8 Positioning of the forearm. Cranio-caudal.

■ *Objective*
To image the forearm, including the elbow and carpal joints.

■ *Central ray of the primary beam*
Direct the x-ray beam perpendicular to the cassette, centered in the middle of the radius.

■ *Notice*
Stretch both limbs cranially; extend the head and neck dorsally; only the caudal border of olecranon touches the cassette; do not tilt!

3 Schultergliedmaße – Thoracic limb

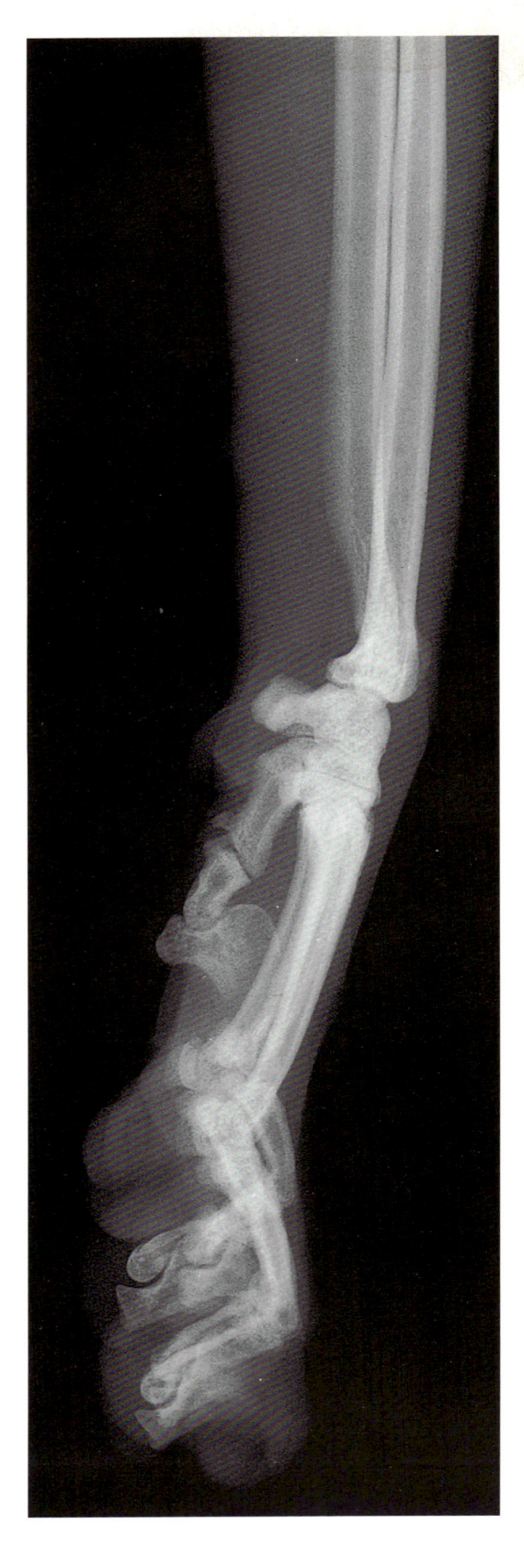

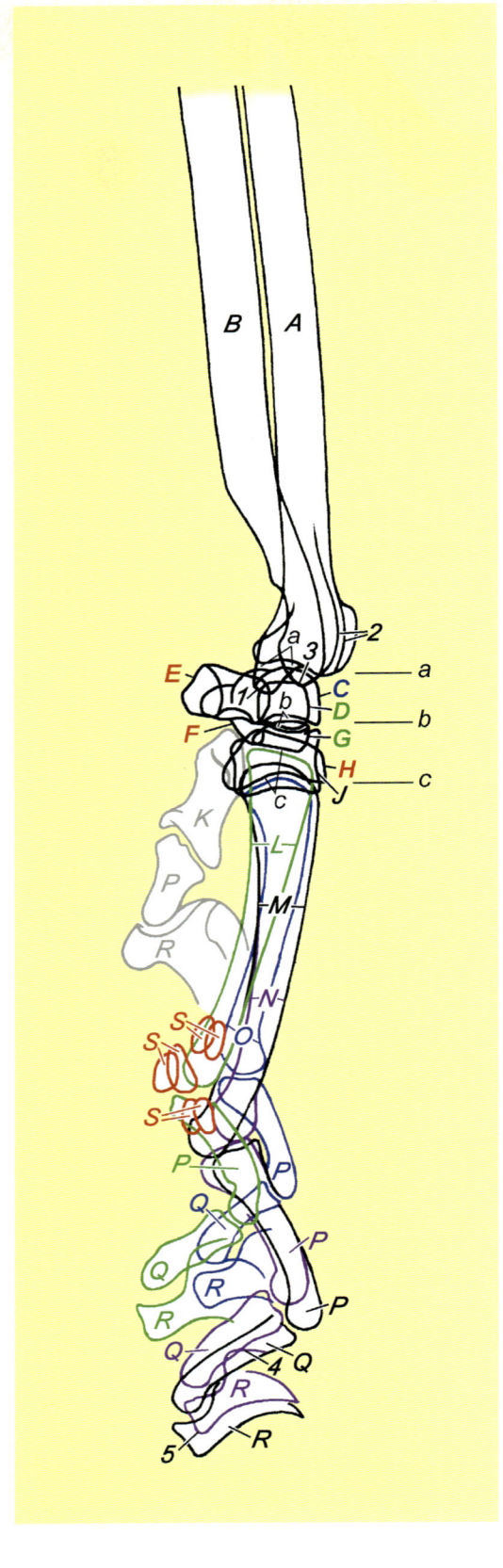

Abb. 3.9 Linker Vorderfuß,
medio-lateral,
Katze
(Ausschnitt aus 13 × 18 cm)

***Fig. 3.9** Left forepaw,
medio-lateral,
Cat
(section of 13 × 18 cm)*

A Radius
  1   Processus styloideus radii
  2   Sehnenrinnen an der Trochlea radii –
       tendon sulci at trochlea radii

B Ulna
  3   Processus styloideus ulnae

C Os carpi intermedioradiale

D Os carpi ulnare

E Os carpi accessorium

F Os carpale I

G Os carpale II

H Os carpale III

J Os carpale IV

K Os metacarpale I

L Os metacarpale II

M Os metacarpale III

N Os metacarpale IV

O Os metacarpale V

P, P, P, P   **Phalanx proximalis**

Q, Q, Q, Q   **Phalanx media**

R, R, R, R, R   **Phalanx distalis**
  4   Crista unguicularis (Digitus IV)
  5   Tuberculum flexorium (Digitus IV)

S Ossa sesamoidea proximalia

a Articulatio antebrachiocarpea

b Articulatio mediocarpea

c Articulationes carpometacarpeae

■ Ziel
Darstellung des Vorderfußes sowie der gelenknahen Abschnitte von Radius und Ulna.

■ Zentralstrahl
Senkrecht zur Kassette, medial in Höhe des Karpalgelenks.

■ Beachte
Unten liegende (zu untersuchende) Gliedmaße distal strecken, während die oben liegende Gliedmaße nach hinten verlagert wird; Kopf und Hals nach dorsal strecken. Pfote nicht supinieren!

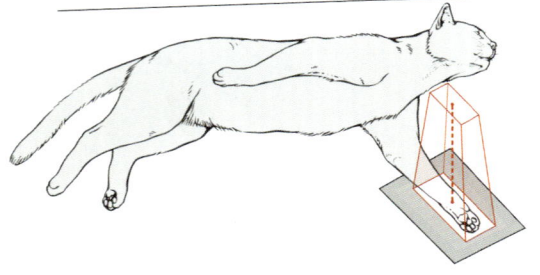

Abb. 3.9 Lagerung zur Aufnahme des Karpalgelenks. Medio-lateral.

***Fig. 3.9** Positioning of the carpal joint. Medio-lateral.*

■ *Objective*
To image the forepaw and adjacent parts of the radius and ulna.

■ *Central ray of the primary beam*
Direct the x-ray beam perpendicular to the cassette, centered at the level of the carpus.

■ *Notice*
The patient lies on the side of interest, stretch the dependent limb distally and the nondependent limb caudally to the dependent stifle; extend the head and neck dorsally, do not supinate the forepaw!

3.10 Rechter Vorderfuß – Right forepaw ■ dorso-palmar

A Radius
 1 Processus styloideus radii
 2 Begrenzung einer dorsalen Sehnenrinne – *border of the tendon sulcus*

B Ulna
 3 Processus styloideus ulnae

C Os carpi intermedioradiale

D Os carpi ulnare

E Os carpi accessorium

F Os carpale I

G Os carpale II

H Os carpale III

J Os carpale IV

K Os metacarpale I

L Os metacarpale II

M Os metacarpale III

N Os metacarpale IV

O Os metacarpale V

P Phalanx proximalis

Q Phalanx media

R Phalanx distalis
 4 Crista unguicularis
 5 Tuberculum flexorium

S Ossa sesamoidea proximalia

T Os sesamoideum m. abductoris pollicis longi

a Articulatio antebrachiocarpea

b Articulatio mediocarpea

c Articulationes carpometacarpeae

d Articulatio metacarpophalangea

e Articulatio interphalangea proximalis manus

f Articulatio interphalangea distalis manus

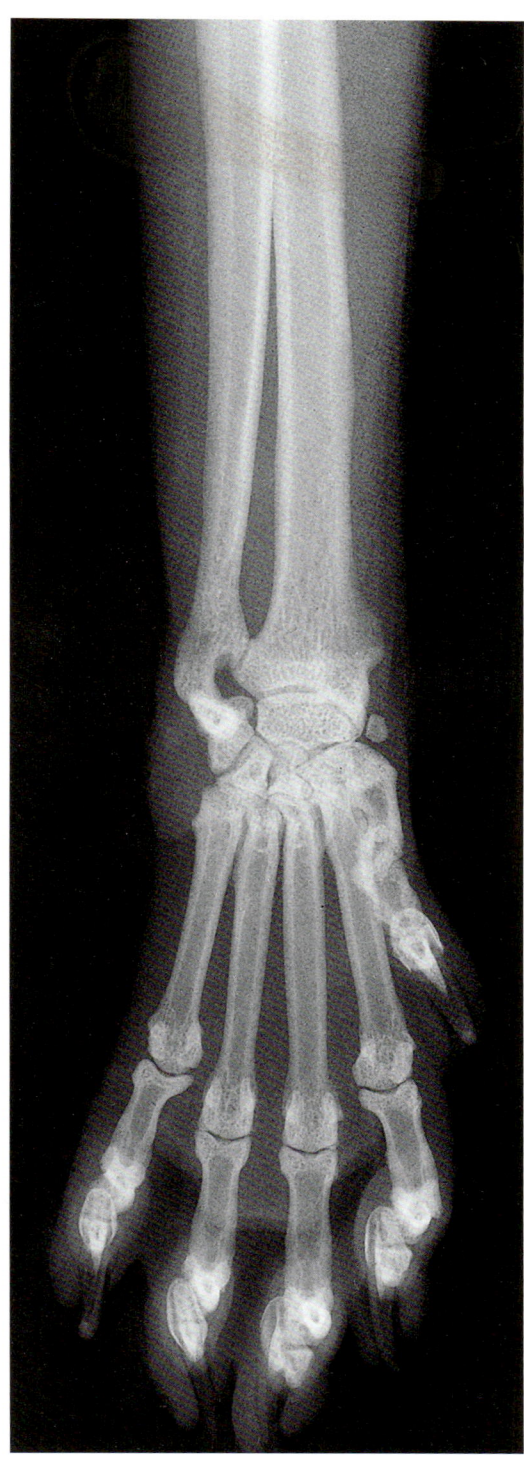

Abb. 3.10 Rechter Vorderfuß, dorso-palmar, Katze
(Ausschnitt aus 13 × 18 cm)

Fig. 3.10 Right forepaw, dorso-palmar, Cat
(section of 13 × 18 cm)

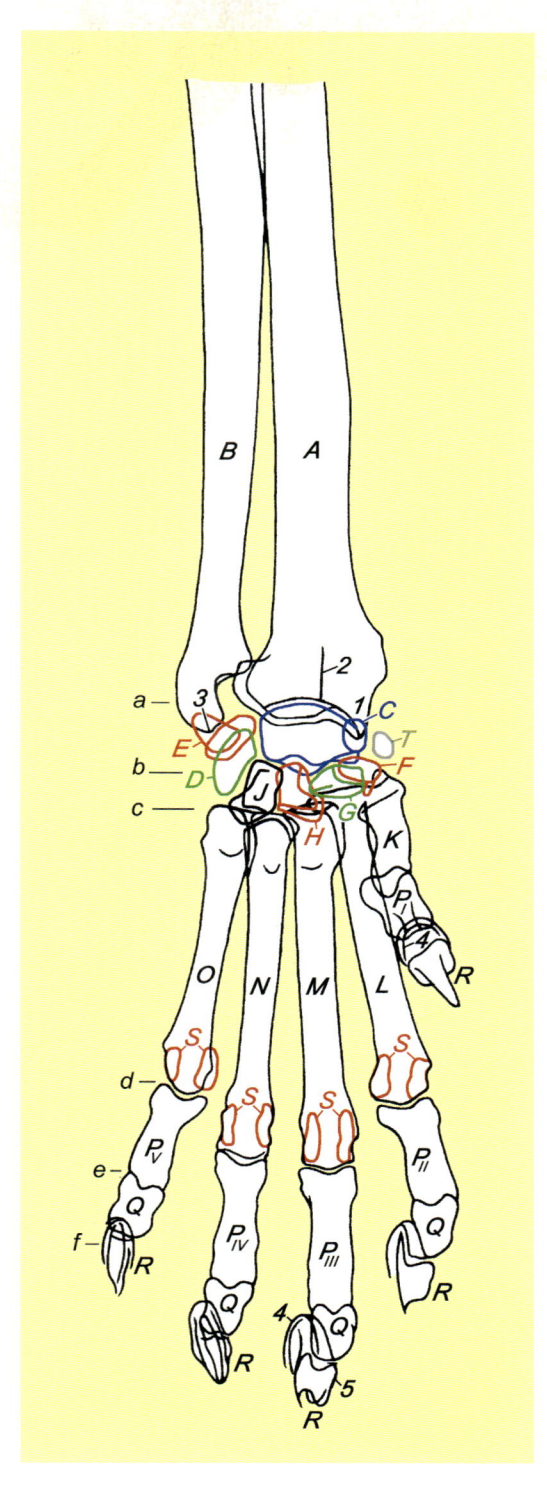

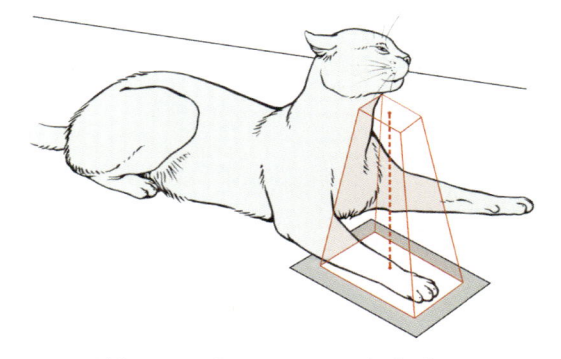

Abb. 3.10 Lagerung zur Aufnahme der Vorderfuß. Dorso-palmar.

Fig. 3.10 Positioning of the forepaw. Dorso-palmar.

■ **Ziel**
Darstellung des Vorderfußes sowie der gelenknahen Abschnitte von Radius und Ulna.

■ **Zentralstrahl**
Senkrecht zur Kassette, dorsal in Höhe des Karpalgelenks.

■ **Beachte**
Kopf und Hals nach dorsal strecken; Schultergliedmaße im Ellbogen nach vorn strecken. Pfote nicht supinieren!

■ *Objective*
To image the forepaw and adjacent parts of the radius and ulna.

■ *Central ray of the primary beam*
Direct the x-ray beam perpendicular to the cassette, centered at the level of the carpus.

■ *Notice*
Extend head and neck dorsally and stretch the thoracic limb and the elbow joint cranially, do not supinate the forepaw!

Tabelle 3.1 Zeitliches Auftreten der Ossifikationspunkte sowie des Apo- und Epiphysenfugenschlusses am Skelett der Schultergliedmaße der Hauskatze (nach I. Horvath, 1983)

Table 3.1 Time-table of the appearance of ossification centers and closures of apo- and epiphyseal lines of the thoracic limb in the domestic cat (after I. Horvath, 1983)

Ossifikationspunkte Apo- und Epiphysen / *Ossification centers Apophyses and Epiphyses*	Auftreten der Ossifikationspunkte (Angabe in Tagen) / *Appearance of the ossification centers (in days)*	Apo- und Epiphysenfugenschluss (Angabe in Monaten) / *Fusion of epi- and apophyseal lines (in months)*
SCAPULA		
Tuberculum supraglenoidale	49–84	5–6
Processus coracoideus	49–84	5–6
HUMERUS		
Epiphysis proximalis humeri	8–14	22–24
Tuberculum minus	70–113	4–7
Condylus humeri		
Capitulum (lateral)	13–21	4–7*
Trochlea (medial)	28–36	5–7*
Epicondylus medialis humeri	49–64	4–6
Epicondylus lateralis humeri	49–73	5–7
RADIUS		
Epiphysis proximalis radii	20–28	5–7
Epiphysis distalis radii	20–24	19–25
ULNA		
Apophysis (proximalis) ulnae	34–38	12–14
Epiphysis distalis ulnae	21–31	19–22
OSSA CARPI		
Os carpi radiale	29–43	
Os carpi intermedium	22–36	
Os carpi centrale	20–24	
Os carpi ulnare	29–42	
Os carpi accessorium	20–28	6–7**
Apophysis ossis carpi accessorii	42–59	
Os carpale I	22–35	
Os carpale II, III	20–28	
Os carpale IV	20–29	
OSSA METACARPALIA		
Epiphysis proximalis ossis metacarpalis I	29–42	9–11
Epiphyses distales ossium metacarpalium II, III, IV, V	20–29	10–12
OSSA DIGITORUM MANUS		
Epiphysis proximalis		
– phalangis proximalis I	29–42	7–9
– phalangium proximalium II, III, IV	20–28	7–9
– phalangis proximalis V	27–36	7–9
– phalangium mediarum II, V	22–35	6–9
– phalangium mediarum III, IV	20–35	6–9
OSSA SESAMOIDEA		
Os sesamoideum proximale digiti I	102–156	
Ossa sesamoidea proximalia digitorum II, V	63–113	
Ossa sesamoidea proximalia digitorum III, IV	63–100	
Os sesamoideum m. abductoris pollicis longi	99–183	

* Fusion von Ossifikationskernen, kurz vor dem Apo- bzw. Epiphysenfugenschluss – *fusion of ossification centers shortly before the fusion of apo- or epiphyseal lines*
** Fusion von Ossifikationskernen – *fusion of ossification centers*

3 Schultergliedmaße – Thoracic limb

Abb. 3.11 Postnatale Entwicklung, rechtes Schultergelenk, medio-lateral, Katze, Lebensalter in Tagen (d)

Abb. 3.12 Postnatale Entwicklung, linkes Schultergelenk, kaudo-kranial, Katze, Lebensalter in Tagen (d)

Fig. 3.11 Postnatal development, right shoulder joint, medio-lateral, Cat, age in days (d)

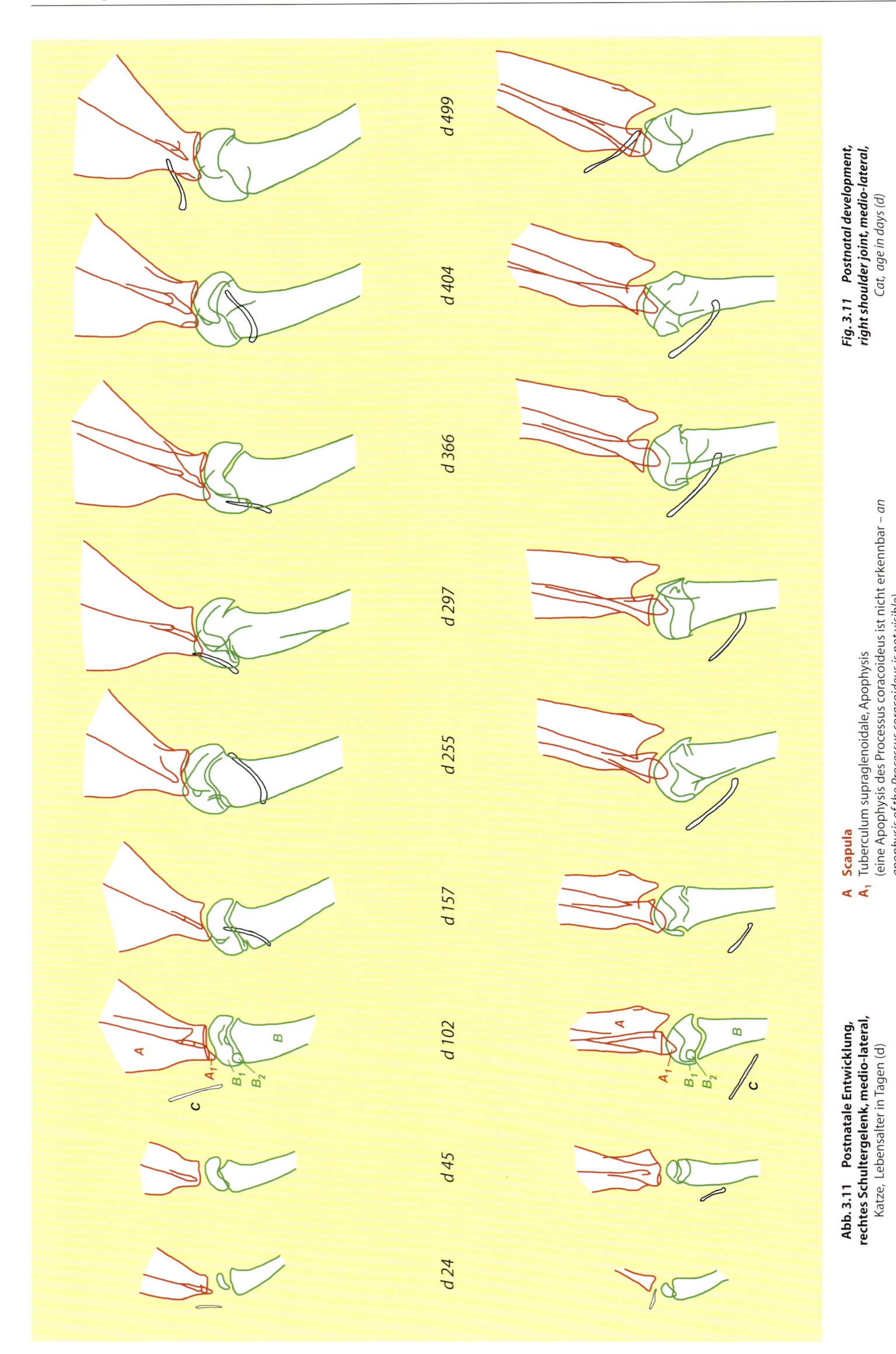

Fig. 3.12 Postnatal development, left shoulder joint, caudo-cranial, Cat, age in days (d)

A Scapula
A₁ Tuberculum supraglenoidale, Apophysis (eine Apophysis des Processus coracoideus ist nicht erkennbar – *an apophysis of the Processus coracoideus is not visible*)

B Humerus
B₁ Caput humeri et Tuberculum majus, Epiphysis proximalis
B₂ Tuberculum minus, Apophysis

C Clavicula

3.13/3.14 Postnatale Entwicklung – Postnatal development ■ rechtes Ellbogengelenk – right elbow joint

d 499   d 404   d 366   d 297   d 255   d 157   d 102   d 45   d 24

Abb. 3.13 Postnatale Entwicklung, rechtes Ellbogengelenk, medio-lateral, Katze, Lebensalter in Tagen (d)

Abb. 3.14 Postnatale Entwicklung, rechtes Ellbogengelenk, kranio-kaudal, Katze, Lebensalter in Tagen (d)

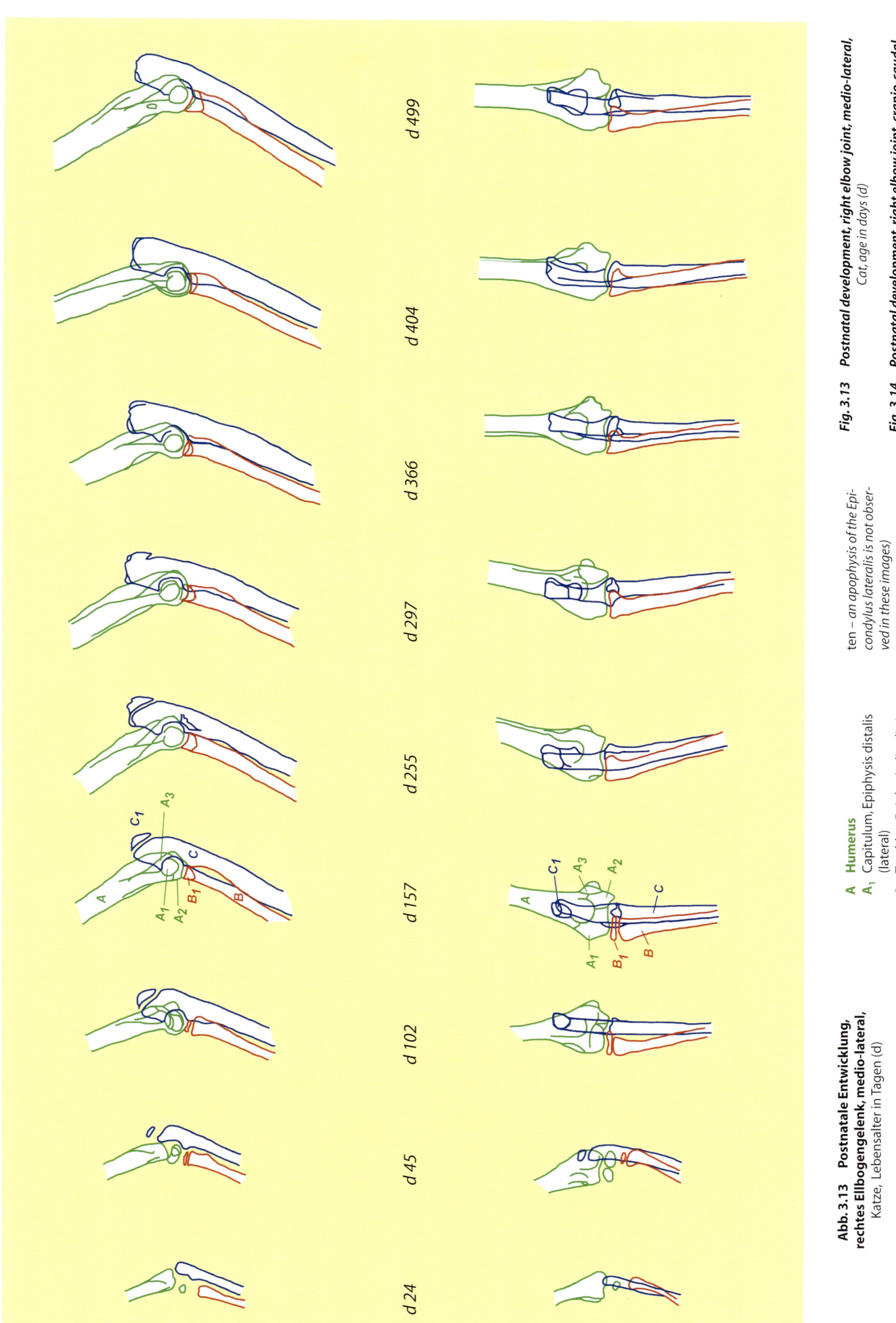

Fig. 3.13 Postnatal development, right elbow joint, medio-lateral, Cat, age in days (d)

Fig. 3.14 Postnatal development, right elbow joint, cranio-caudal, Cat, age in days (d)

A Humerus
A_1 Capitulum, Epiphysis distalis (lateral)
A_2 Trochlea, Epiphysis distalis (medial)
A_3 Epicondylus medialis, Apophysis (eine Apophyse für den Epicondylus lateralis ist in den Aufnahmen nicht zu beobachten – an apophysis of the Epicondylus lateralis is not observed in these images)

B Radius
B_1 Caput, Epiphysis proximalis

C Ulna
C_1 Tuber olecrani, Apophysis

55

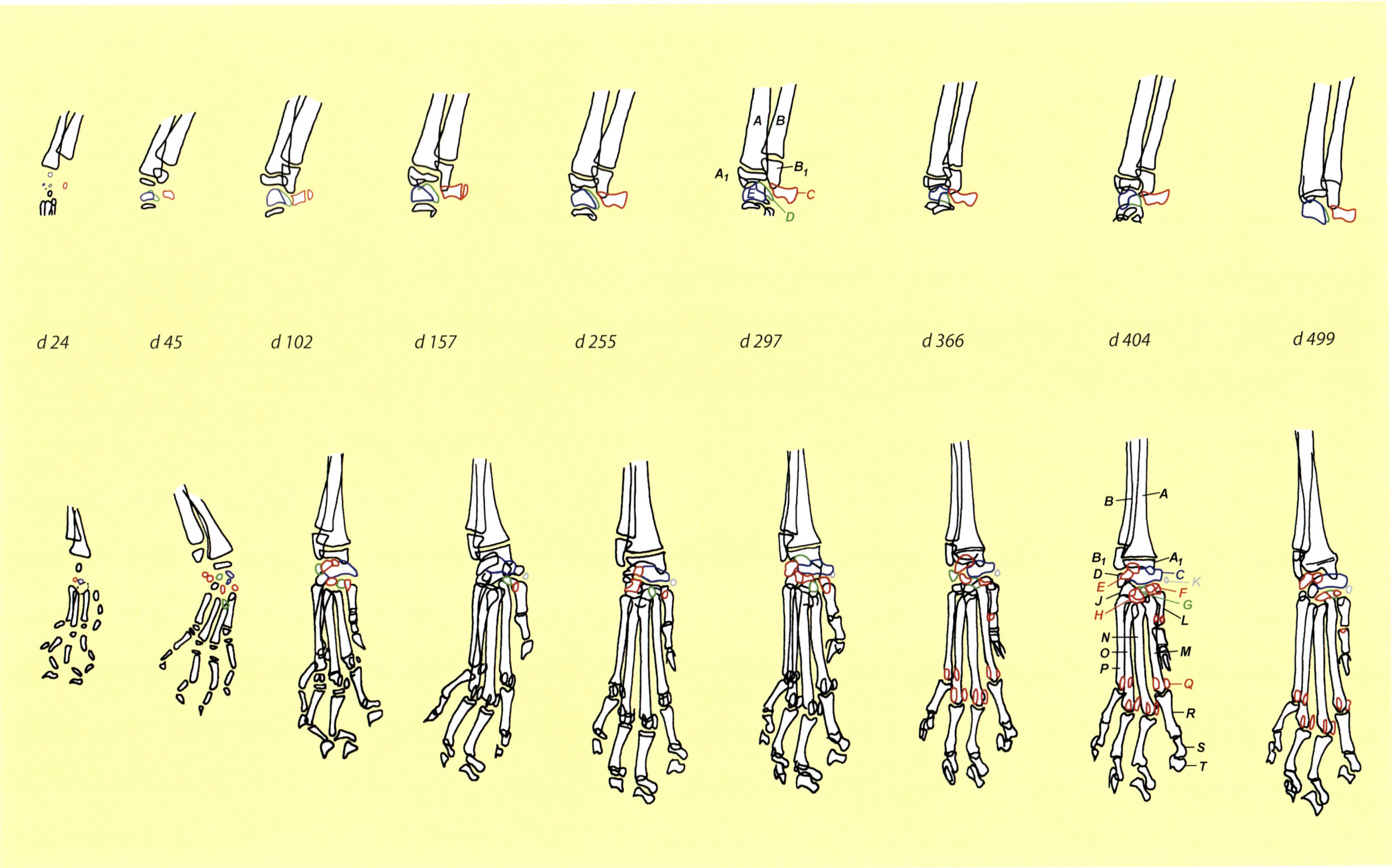

3 Schultergliedmaße – Thoracic limb

Abb. 3.15 Postnatale Entwicklung, rechtes Karpalgelenk, medio-lateral,
Katze, Lebensalter in Tagen (d)

Fig. 3.15 Postnatal development, right carpal joint, medio-lateral,
Cat, age in days (d)

Abb. 3.16 Postnatale Entwicklung, rechter Vorderfuß, dorso-palmar,
Katze, Lebensalter in Tagen (d)

Fig. 3.16 Postnatal development, right forepaw, dorso-palmar,
Cat, age in days (d)

3.15/3.16 Postnatale Entwicklung – Postnatal development ■ rechtes Karpalgelenk – right carpal joint

A **Radius**
A₁ Trochlea radii, Epiphysis distalis

B **Ulna**
B₁ Caput ulnae, Epiphysis

C **Os carpi intermedioradiale**

D **Os carpi ulnare**

E **Os carpi accessorium**

F **Os carpale I**

G **Os carpale II**

H **Os carpale III**

J **Os carpale IV**

K Os sesamoideum m. abductoris pollicis longi

L **Os metacarpale I**

M **Os metacarpale II**

N **Os metacarpale III**

O **Os metacarpale IV**

P **Os metacarpale V**

Q **Ossa sesamoidea proximalia, Digiti II–V, Digitus I, unpaar –** *impair*

R **Phalanx proximalis, Digiti I–V**

S **Phalanx media, Digiti II–V**

T **Phalanx distalis**

4 Beckengliedmaße – Pelvic limb

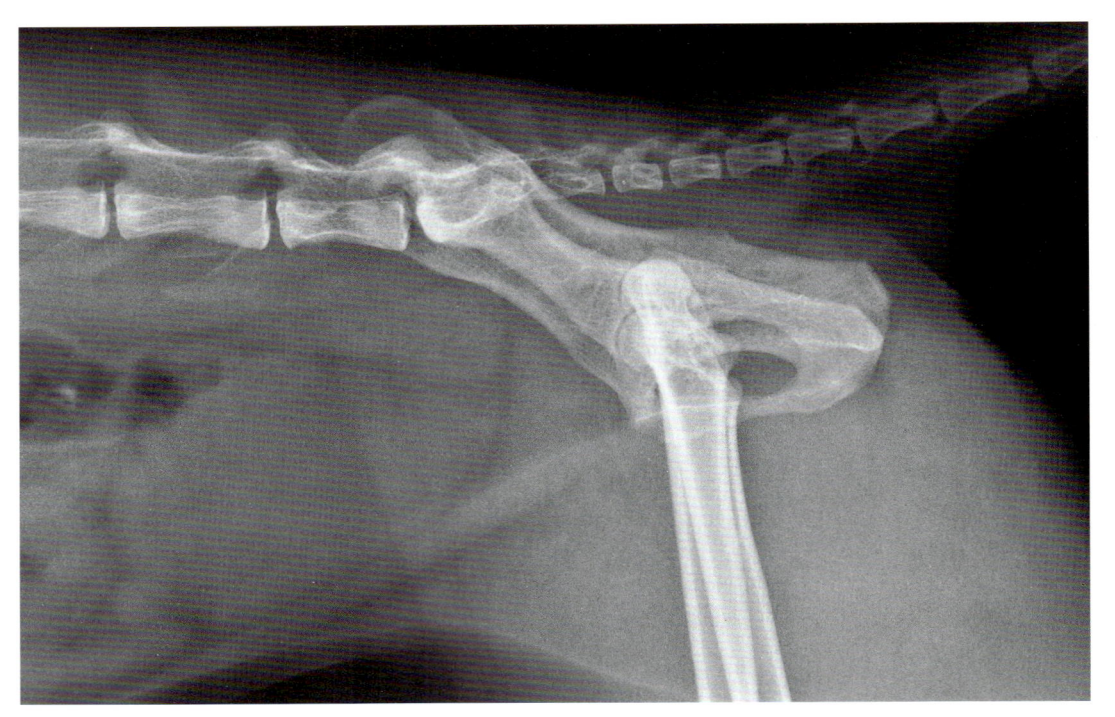

**Abb. 4.1 Becken,
latero-lateral,**
Katze
(Ausschnitt aus 18 × 24 cm)

*Fig. 4.1 Pelvis,
latero-lateral,*
Cat
(section of 18 × 24 cm)

■ Ziel
Laterale Darstellung des Beckens.

■ Zentralstrahl
Senkrecht zur Kassette, auf den Trochanter major der oben liegenden Gliedmaße.

■ Beachte
Leicht gestreckte Beckengliedmaßen, bei adipösen Tieren sind die Gliedmaßen durch Schaumgummikeile zu unterlegen; der Schwanz sollte nach kaudo-dorsal fixiert sein.

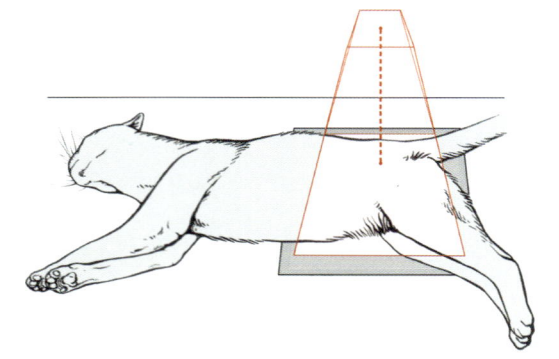

**Abb. 4.1   Lagerung zur Aufnahme des
Beckens. Latero-lateral.**

*Fig. 4.1   Positioning of the pelvis.
Latero-lateral.*

■ *Objective*
To obtain a lateral radiograph of the pelvis.

■ *Central ray of the primary beam*
Direct the x-ray beam perpendicular to the cassette, with the central ray centered on the greater trochanter of the nondependent limb.

■ *Notice*
Stretch the pelvic limbs slightly, support the limbs with foam rubber wedges in obese cats, fix the tail caudo-dorsally.

4.1 Becken – Pelvis ■ latero-lateral

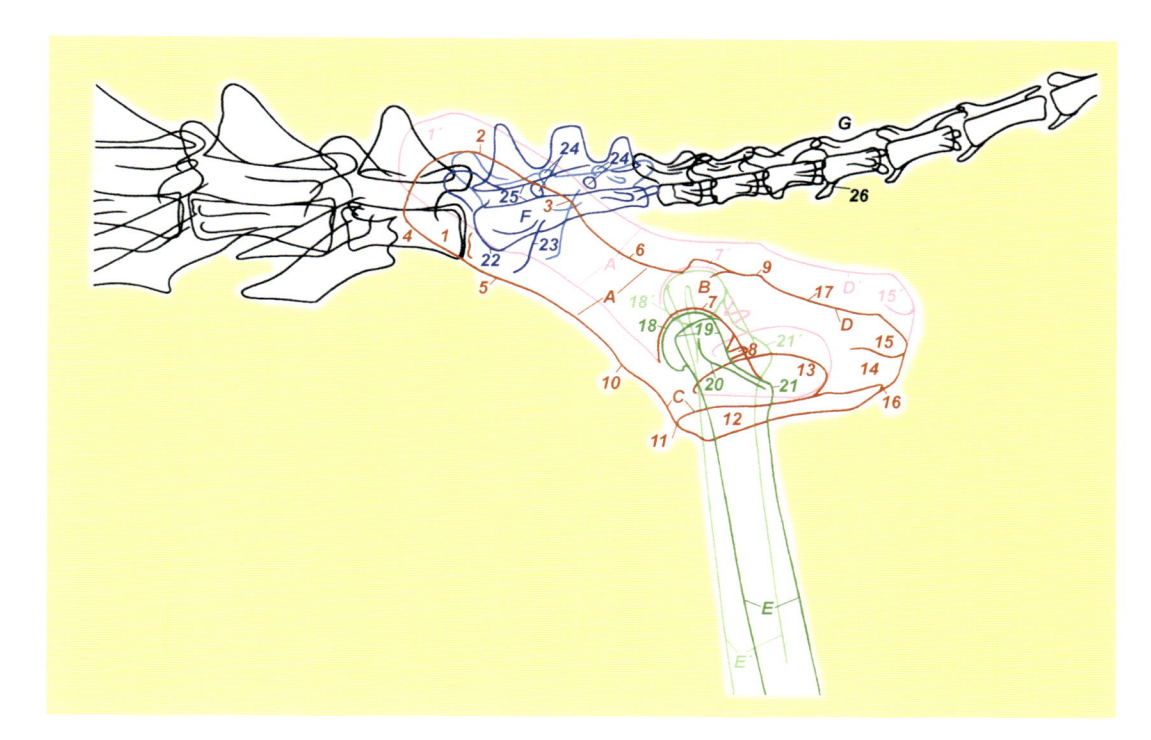

A Os ilium, A´ plattenfern – *next to the tube*
 1 Ala ossi ilii, 1´ plattenfern – *next to the tube*
 2 Tuber sacrale, Spina iliaca dorsalis cranialis
 3 Tuber sacrale, Spina iliaca dorsalis caudalis
 4 Tuber coxae, Spina iliaca ventralis cranialis
 5 Spina alaris
 6 Incisura ischiadica major

B Os coxae
 7 Acetabulum, 7´ plattenfern – *next to the tube*
 8 Incisura acetabuli
 9 Spina ischiadica

C Os pubis
 10 Eminentia iliopubica
 11 Pecten ossis pubis
 12 Symphysis pelvina

D Os ischii, D´ plattenfern – *next to the tube*
 13 Foramen obturatum
 14 Tabula ossis ischii
 15 Tuber ischiadicum, 15´ plattenfern – *next to the tube*
 16 Arcus ischiadicus
 17 Incisura ischiadica minor

E Os femoris, E´ plattenfern – *next to the tube*
 18 Caput ossis femoris, 18´ plattenfern – *next to the tube*
 19 Trochanter major
 20 Fossa trochanterica
 21 Trochanter minor, 21´ plattenfern – *next to the tube*

F Os sacrum
 22 Promontorium
 23 Ala ossis sacri, kaudaler Rand – *caudal border*
 24 Foramina sacralia dorsalia
 25 Canalis sacralis

G Co IV
 26 Processus haemalis

4 Beckengliedmaße – Pelvic limb

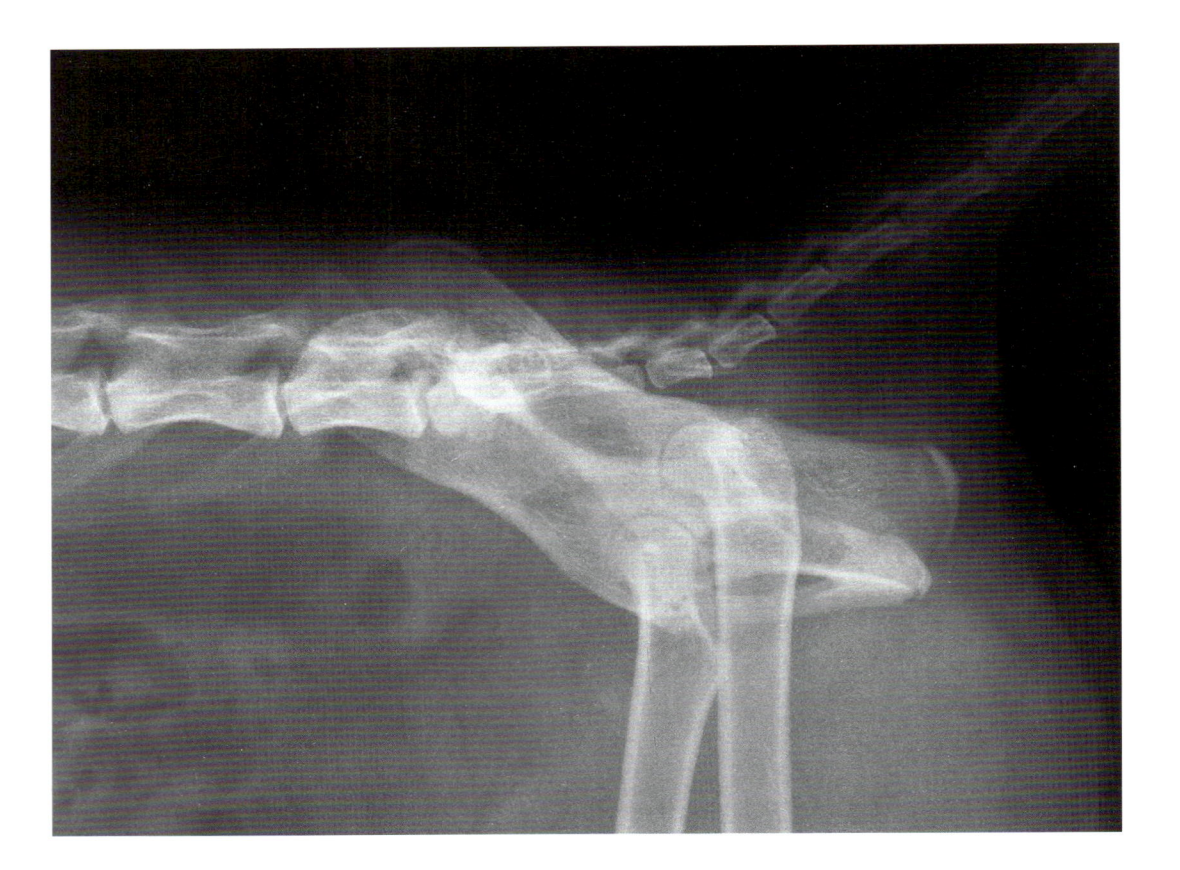

**Abb. 4.2 Becken, latero-lateral,
Schrägprojektion (20°)**
Katze
(Ausschnitt aus 18 × 24 cm)

*Fig. 4.2 Pelvis, obliquely
latero-lateral (20°),*
Cat
(section of 18 × 24 cm)

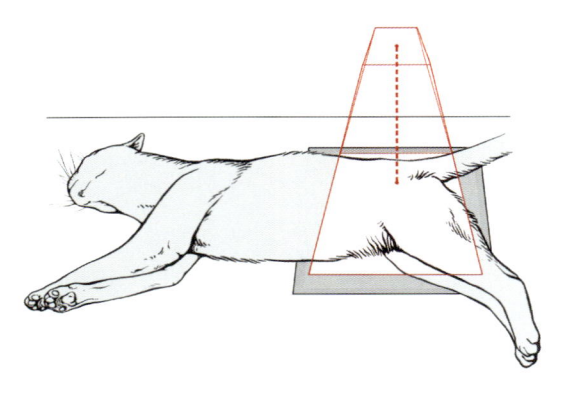

■ **Ziel**
Getrennte Darstellung beider Beckenhälften von lateral (rot plattennahe; rosa plattenferne Seite).

■ **Zentralstrahl**
Senkrecht zur Kassette, fingerbreit dorsal des Trochanter major der oben liegenden Gliedmaße.

■ **Beachte**
Kippung des Beckens um 20° durch Unterlegen eines Schaumgummikeils, leicht gestreckte Beckengliedmaßen, der Schwanz sollte nach kaudo-dorsal fixiert sein.

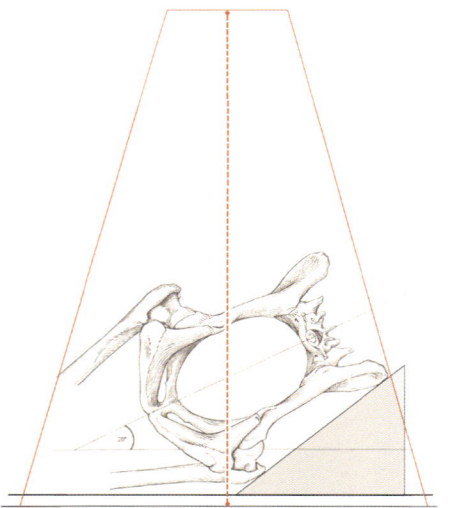

**Abb. 4.2 Lagerung zur Aufnahme des
Beckens. Latero-lateral. Schrägaufnahme.**

*Fig. 4.2 Positioning of the pelvis.
Latero-lateral. Oblique.*

■ *Objective*
To obtain a lateral radiograph of the dependent hemipelvis without superimposition of the opposite side (red near to the cassette, pink near to the tube).

■ *Central ray of the primary beam*
Direct the x-ray beam perpendicular to the cassette, with the central ray centered one finger width dorsal to the greater trochanter of the nondependent limb.

■ *Notice*
Use a foam rubber wedge to rotate the pelvis about 20 degrees, stretch the pelvic limbs slightly, fix the tail caudo-dorsally.

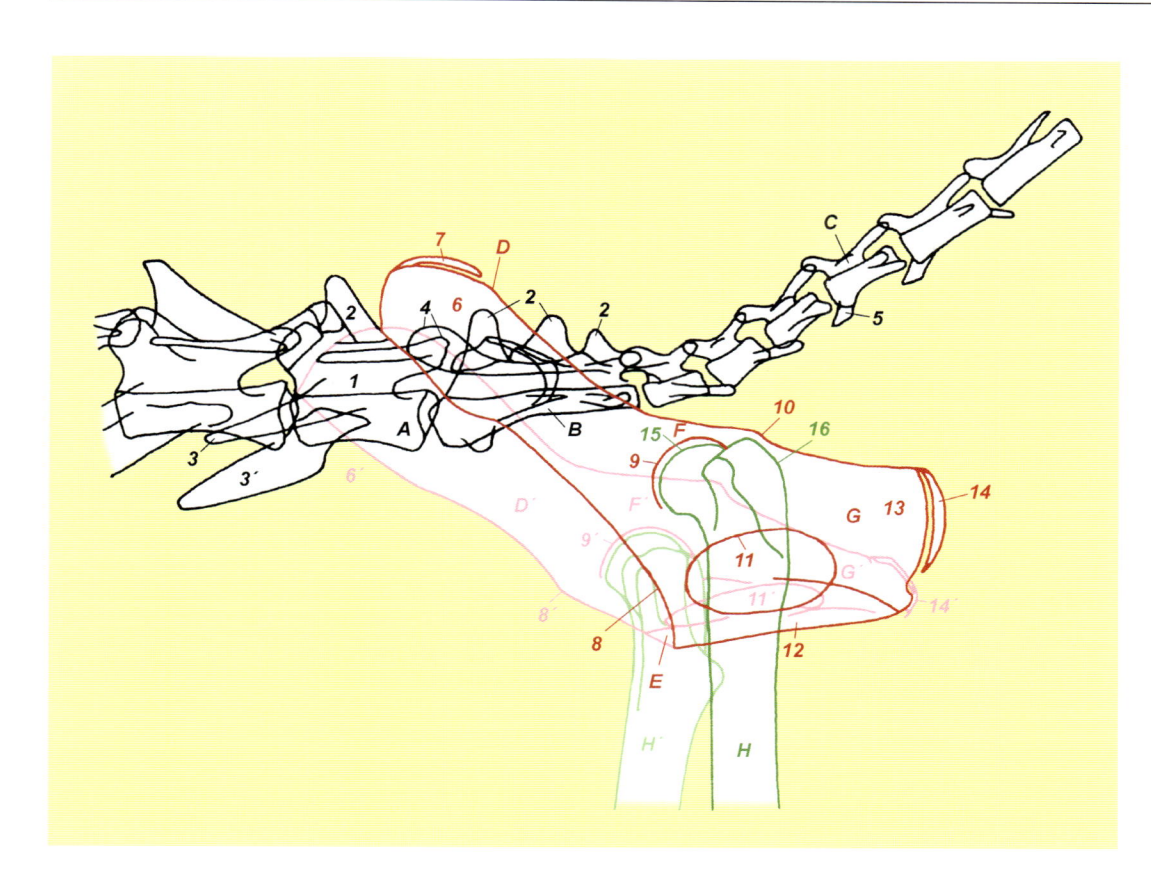

4.2 Becken – Pelvis ◼ latero-lateral

A L VII
  1 Canalis vertebralis
  2 Processus spinosus
  3 Processus transversus, 3´ plattenfern – *next to the tube*

B Os sacrum
  2 Processus spinosus
  4 Processus articulares caudales (LVII) et craniales (Os sacrum)

C Co IV
  5 Processus haemalis

D Os ilium, D´ plattenfern – *next to the tube*
  6 Ala ossi ilii, 6´ plattenfern – *next to the tube*
  7 Crista iliaca, Apophysis der Spina iliaca dorsalis cranialis – *Apophysis of the dorsal cranial iliac spine*

E Os pubis
  8 Eminentia iliopubica, 8´ plattenfern – *next to the tube*

F Os coxae, F´ plattenfern – *next to the tube*
  9 Acetabulum, 9´ plattenfern – *next to the tube*
  10 Spina ischiadica

G Os ischii, G´ plattenfern – *next to the tube*
  11 Foramen obturatum, 11´ plattenfern – *next to the tube*
  12 Symphysis pelvina
  13 Tabula ossis ischii
  14 Tuber ischiadicum, Apophysis, 14´ plattenfern – *next to the tube*

H Os femoris, H´ plattenfern – *next to the tube*
  15 Caput ossis femoris
  16 Trochanter major

4 Beckengliedmaße – Pelvic limb

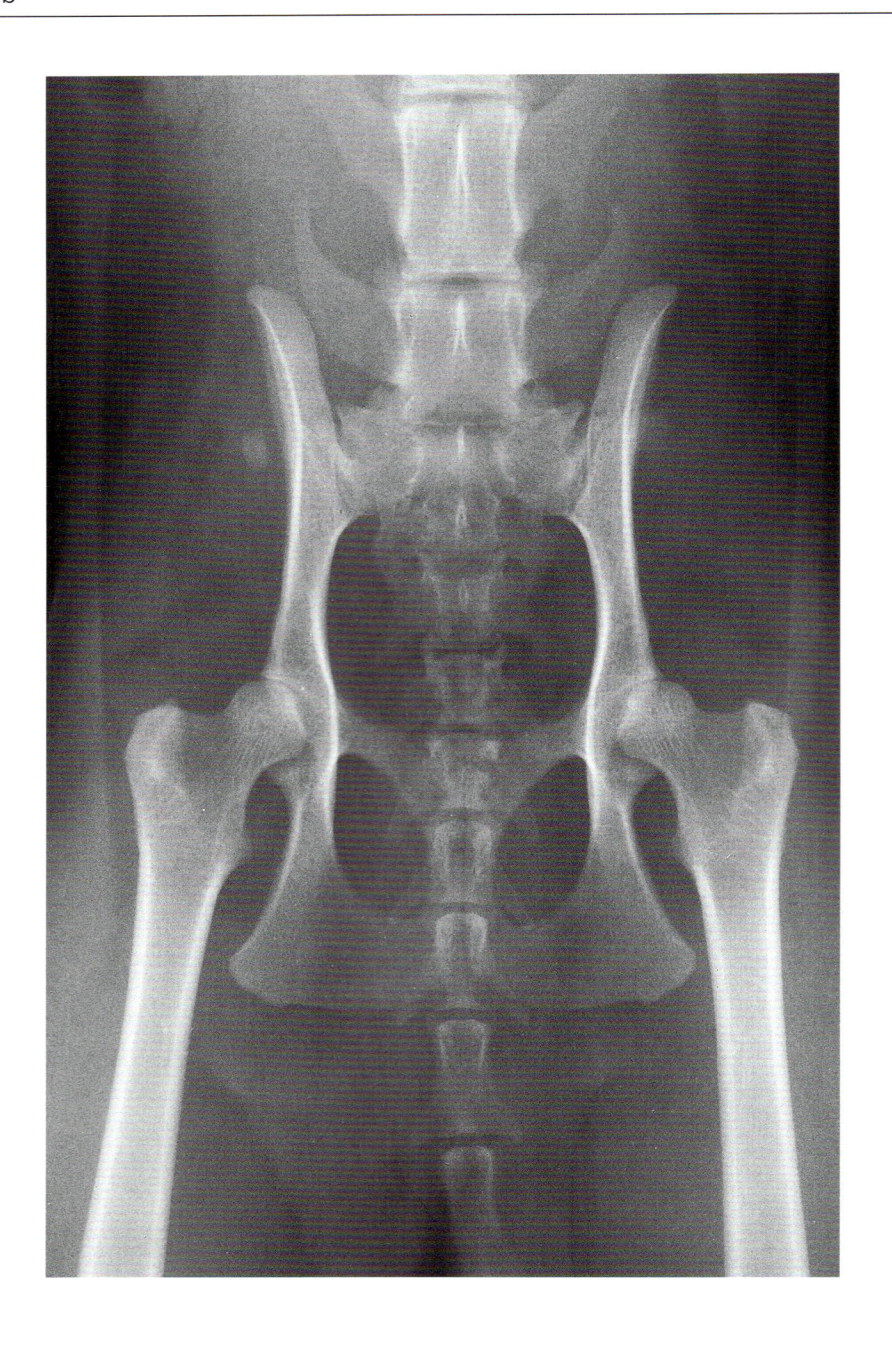

Abb. 4.3 Becken, ventro-dorsal,
Katze
(Ausschnitt aus 18 × 24 cm)

Fig. 4.3 Pelvis, ventro-dorsal,
Cat
(section of 18 × 24 cm)

■ **Ziel**
Symmetrische Darstellung des Beckens und der gestreckten Hüftgelenke in Rückenlage.

■ **Zentralstrahl**
Senkrecht zur Kassette, auf die Verbindungslinie der großen Trochanteren.

■ **Beachte**
Beckengliedmaßen symmetrisch strecken, bis die Sprunggelenke dem Tisch aufliegen.

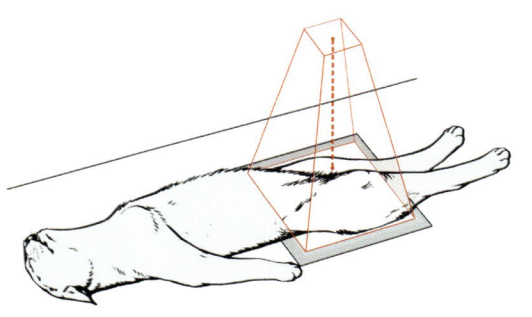

Abb. 4.3 Lagerung zur Aufnahme des Beckens. Ventro-dorsal.

Fig. 4.3 Positioning of the pelvis. Ventro-dorsal.

■ *Objective*
Symmetric view of the pelvis and the stretched hip joints in dorsal recumbency.

■ *Central ray of the primary beam*
Direct the x-ray beam perpendicular to the cassette, with the central ray centered on a line uniting both greater trochanters.

■ *Notice*
Stretch the cat symmetrically in order to prevent rotation along the longitudinal axis.

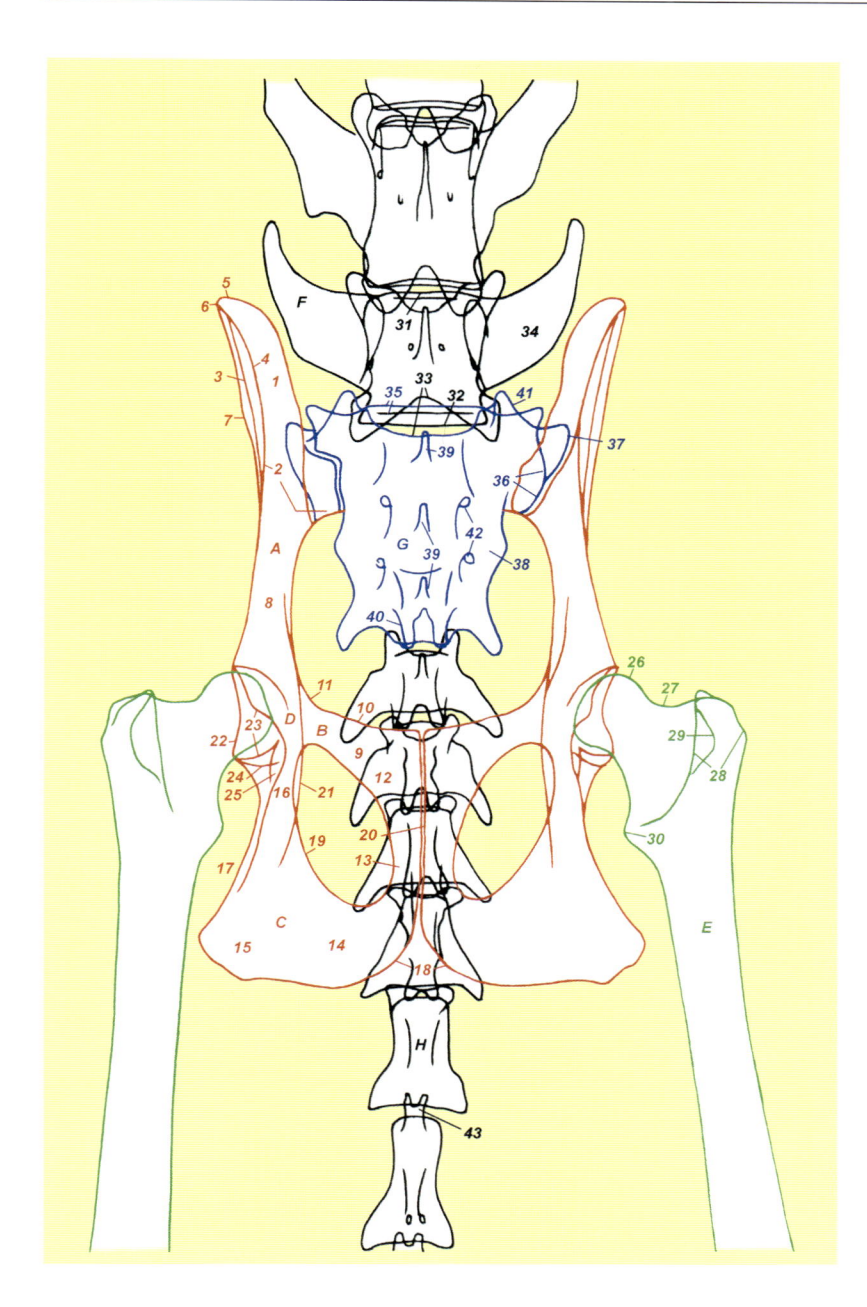

4.3 Becken – Pelvis ◾ ventro-dorsal

A Os ilium
1. Ala ossi ilii
2. Tuber sacrale, Spina iliaca dorsalis caudalis
3. Linea glutaea
4. Facies glutaea
5. Crista iliaca
6. Tuber coxae, Spina iliaca ventralis cranialis
7. Spina alaris
8. Corpus ossis ilii

B Os pubis
9. Ramus cranialis ossis pubis
10. Pecten ossis pubis
11. Eminentia iliopubica
12. Ramus caudalis ossis pubis

C Os ischii
13. Ramus ossis ischii
14. Tabula ossis ischii
15. Tuber ischiadicum
16. Corpus ossis ischii
17. Incisura ischiadica minor
18. Arcus ischiadicus
19. Foramen obturatum
20. Symphysis pelvina

D Os coxae
21. Spina ischiadica
22. Acetabulum, dorsaler Rand – *dorsal border*
23. Acetabulum, ventraler Rand – *ventral border*
24. Facies lunata
25. Incisura acetabuli

E Os femoris
26. Caput ossis femoris
27. Collum ossis femoris
28. Trochanter major
29. Fossa trochanterica
30. Trochanter minor

F L VII
31. Extremitas cranialis
32. Extremitas caudalis
33. Spatium interarcuale lumbosacrale
34. Processus transversus

G Os sacrum
35. Basis ossis sacri
36. Ala ossis sacri, dorsaler Anteil – *dorsal part*
37. Ala ossis sacri, ventraler Anteil – *ventral part*
38. Os sacrum, Pars lateralis
39. Processus spinosus
40. Processus articularis caudalis
41. Processus articularis cranialis
42. Foramina sacralia dorsalia et pelvina, ineinander projiziert – *projected into one another*

H Co V
43. Processus haemalis

4 Beckengliedmaße – Pelvic limb

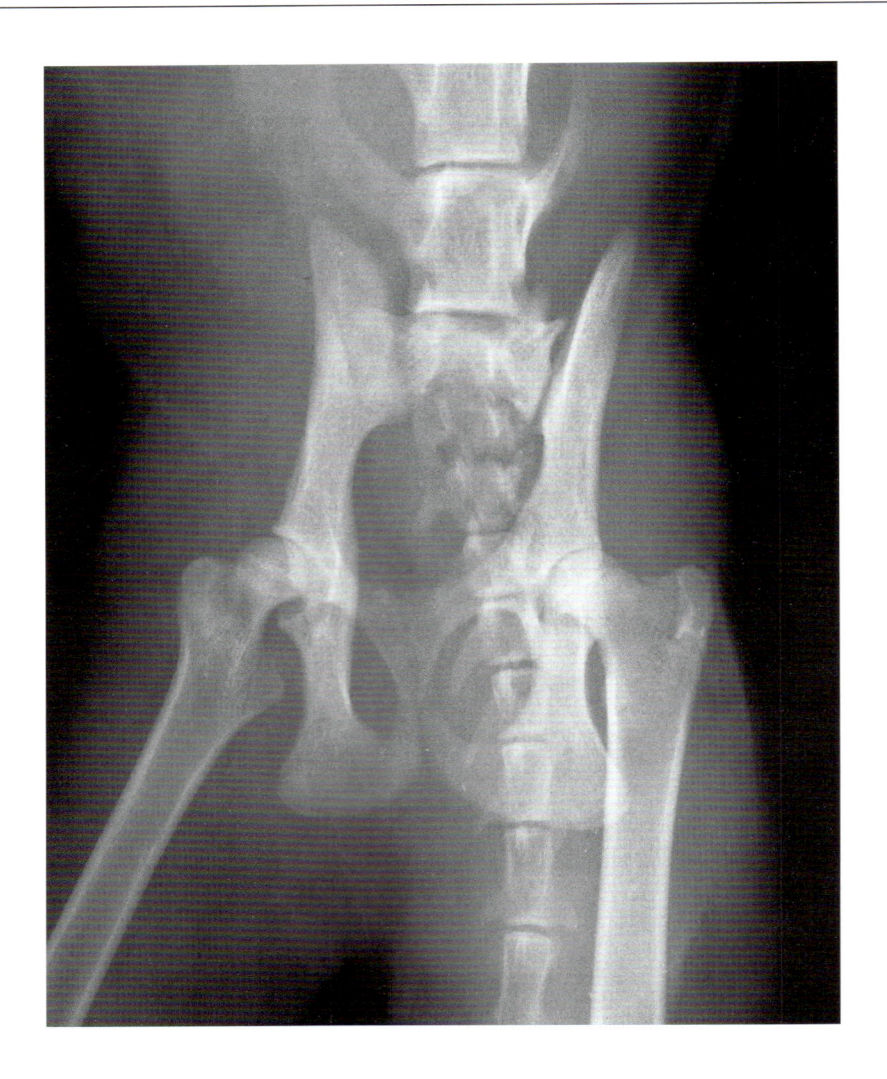

**Abb. 4.4 Becken,
ventro-dorsal, oblique,**
Katze
(Ausschnitt aus 13 × 18 cm)

*Fig. 4.4 Pelvis,
ventro-dorsal, oblique,*
Cat
(section of 13 × 18 cm)

■ **Ziel**
Einseitige Darstellung des Iliosakralgelenks und des zugehörigen dorso-kranialen Randes des Darmbeinflügels in Rückenlage.

■ **Zentralstrahl**
Senkrecht zur Kassette, auf das darzustellende Hüftgelenk.

■ **Beachte**
Leichte Abduktion des gesunden Beines im Hüftgelenk, der Bereich Hüfthöcker, Kreuzbein und Schwanzansatz soll der Unterlage anliegen.

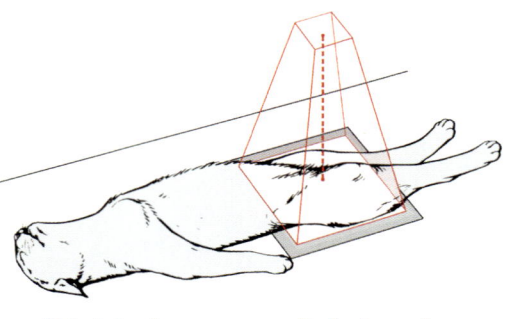

Abb. 4.4 Lagerung zur Aufnahme des Beckens. Ventro-dorsal, oblique.

Fig. 4.4 Positioning of the pelvis. Ventro-dorsal, oblique.

■ *Objective*
To obtain a ventro-dorsal radiograph of one sacroiliac joint and of the adjacent dorso-cranial edge of the wing of the ilium.

■ *Central ray of the primary beam*
Direct the x-ray beam perpendicular to the cassette, with the central ray centered on the dependent coxal joint.

■ *Notice*
Abduct slightly the nondependent pelvic limb, the region of the tuber sacrale, the sacrum and the root of the tail are resting on the supporting surface.

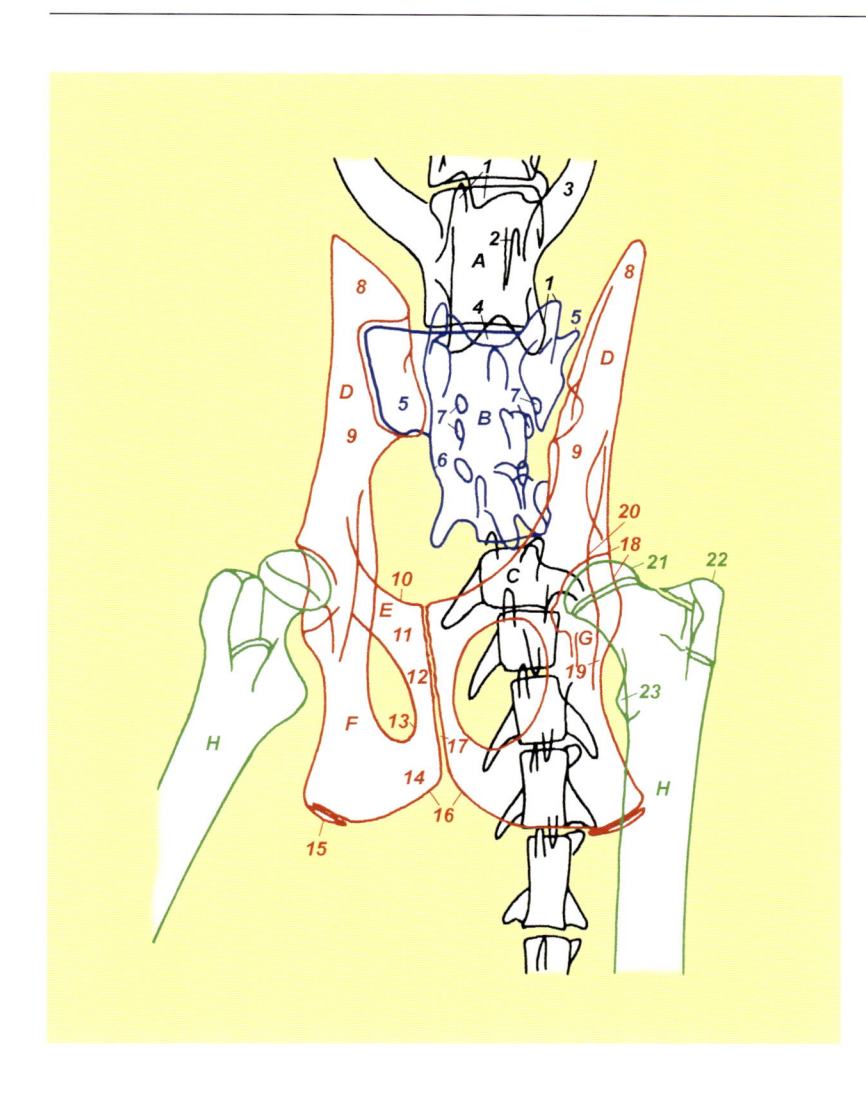

4.4 Becken – Pelvis ■ ventro-dorsal

A L VII
1 Processus articulares caudales (LVII) et craniales (Os sacrum)
2 Processus spinosus
3 Processus transversus
4 Spatium interarcuale lumbosacrale

B Os sacrum
5 Ala sacralis
6 Pars lateralis
7 Foramina sacralia

C Co I

D Os ilium
8 Ala ossis ilii
9 Corpus ossis ilii

E Os pubis
10 Pecten ossis pubis
11 Ramus cranialis ossis pubis
12 Ramus caudalis ossis pubis

F Os ischii
13 Foramen obturatum
14 Tabula ossis ischii
15 Tuber ischiadicum, Apophysis
16 Arcus ischiadicus
17 Symphysis pelvina

G Os coxae
18 Acetabulum
19 Incisura acetabuli
20 Spina ischiadica

H Os femoris
21 Caput ossis femoris, mit Epiphysenfuge – *with epiphyseal plate*
22 Trochanter major, mit Apophysenfuge – *with apophyseal plate*
23 Trochanter minor

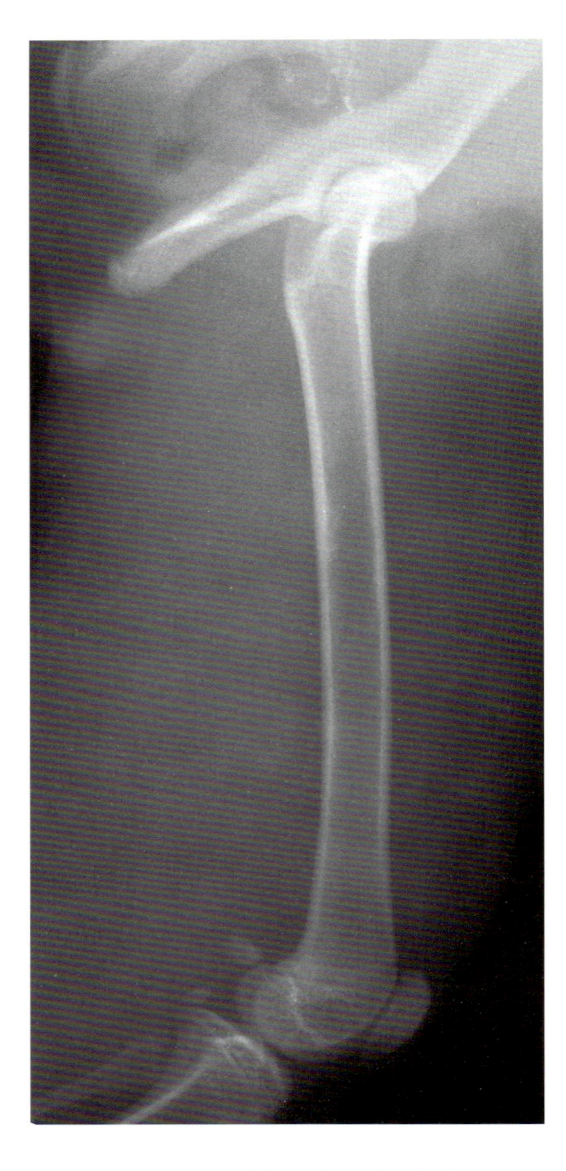

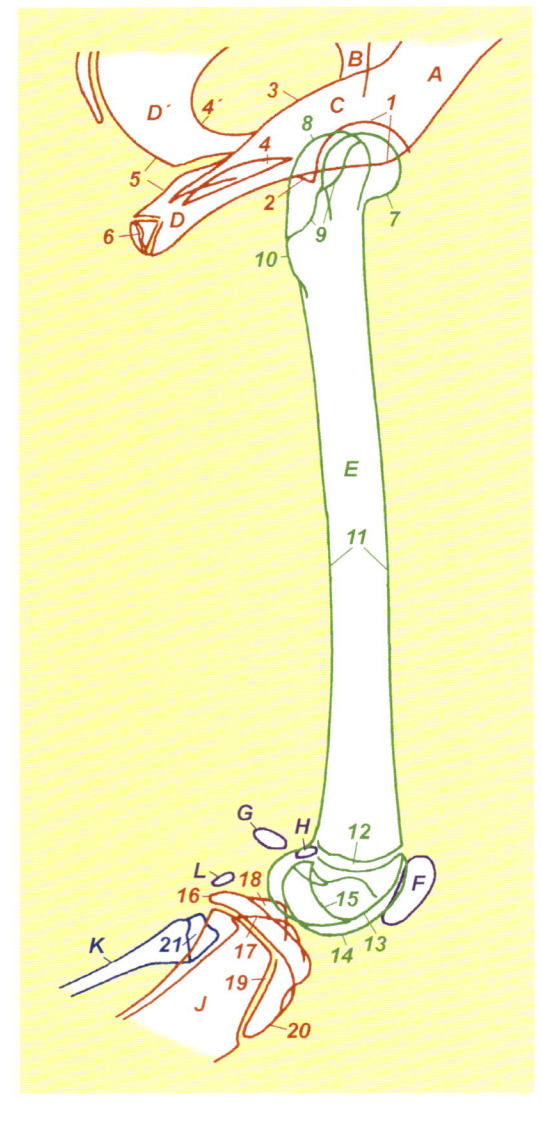

4 Beckengliedmaße – Pelvic limb

A Os ilium

B Os pubis

C Os coxae
  1 Acetabulum
  2 Incisura acetabuli
  3 Spina ischiadica

D Os ischii, D´ plattenfern – *next to the tube*
  4 Foramen obturatum, **4´** plattenfern – *next to the tube*
  5 Arcus ischiadicus
  6 Tuber ischiadicum, Apophysis

E Os femoris
  7 Caput ossis femoris
  8 Trochanter major
  9 Fossa trochanterica
  10 Trochanter minor
  11 Corpus ossis femoris
  12 Cartilago epiphysialis distalis
  13 Condylus lateralis
  14 Condylus medialis
  15 Fossa intercondylaris

F Patella

G Os sesamoideum m. gastrocnemii laterale

H Os sesamoideum m. gastrocnemii mediale

J Tibia
  16 Condylus lateralis
  17 Condylus medialis
  18 Eminentia intercondylaris
  19 Cartilago apophysialis tuberositatis tibiae
  20 Tuberositas tibiae

K Fibula
  21 Caput fibulae, Epiphysis

L Os sesamoideum m. poplitei

Abb. 4.5 Linker Oberschenkel, medio-lateral, Katze
(Ausschnitt aus 13 × 18 cm)

Fig. 4.5 Left thigh, medio-lateral, Cat (section of 13 × 18 cm)

■ **Ziel**
Seitliche Darstellung des Os femoris mit Hüft- und Kniegelenk.

■ **Zentralstrahl**
Senkrecht zur Kassette, medial auf Mitte des Os femoris.

■ **Beachte**
Abduktion der oben liegenden Beckengliedmaße.

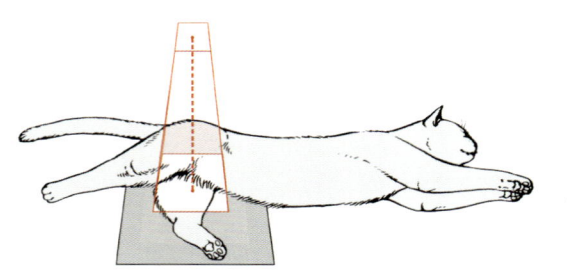

Abb. 4.5 Lagerung zur Aufnahme des Oberschenkels. Medio-lateral.

Fig. 4.5 Positioning of the thigh. Medio-lateral.

■ *Objective*
To obtain a medio-lateral radiograph of the femur, including the hip and stifle joints.

■ *Central ray of the primary beam*
Direct the x-ray beam perpendicular to the cassette, with the central ray centered in the middle of the femur.

■ *Notice*
Abduct the nondependent pelvic limb.

4.6 Linker Oberschenkel – Left thigh ■ kranio-kaudal – cranio-caudal

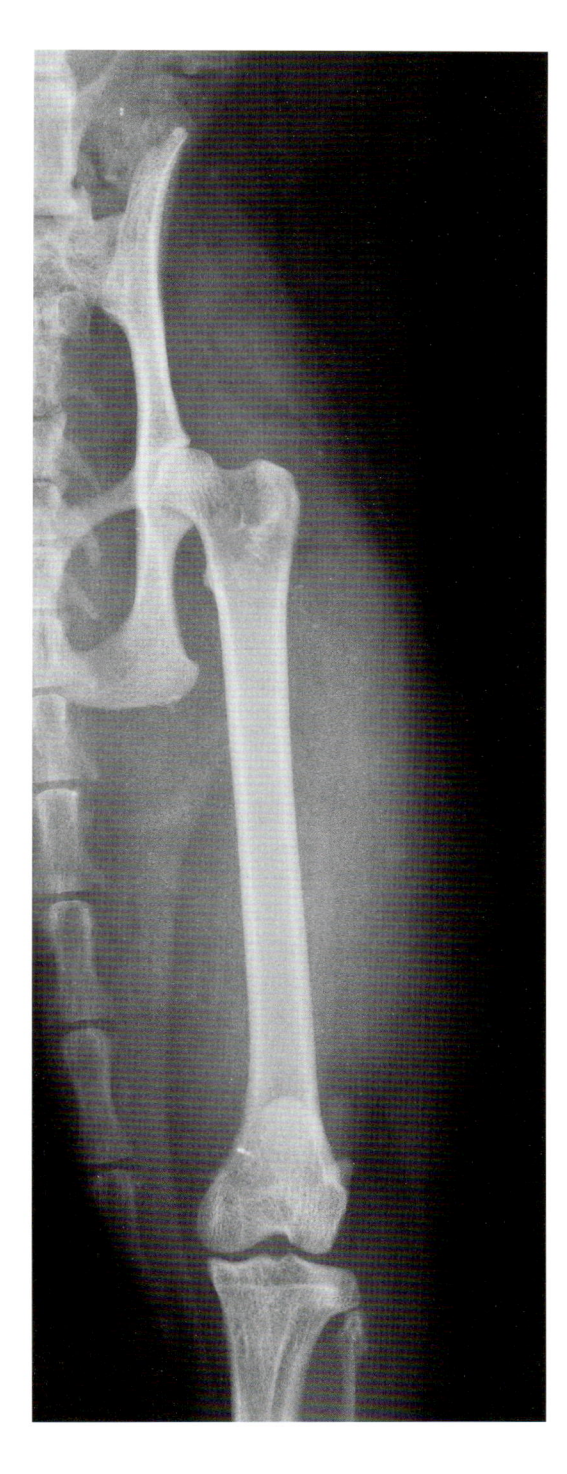

Abb. 4.6 Linker Oberschenkel, kranio-kaudal,
Katze
(Ausschnitt aus 18 × 24 cm)

Fig. 4.6 Left thigh, cranio-caudal,
Cat
(section of 18 × 24 cm)

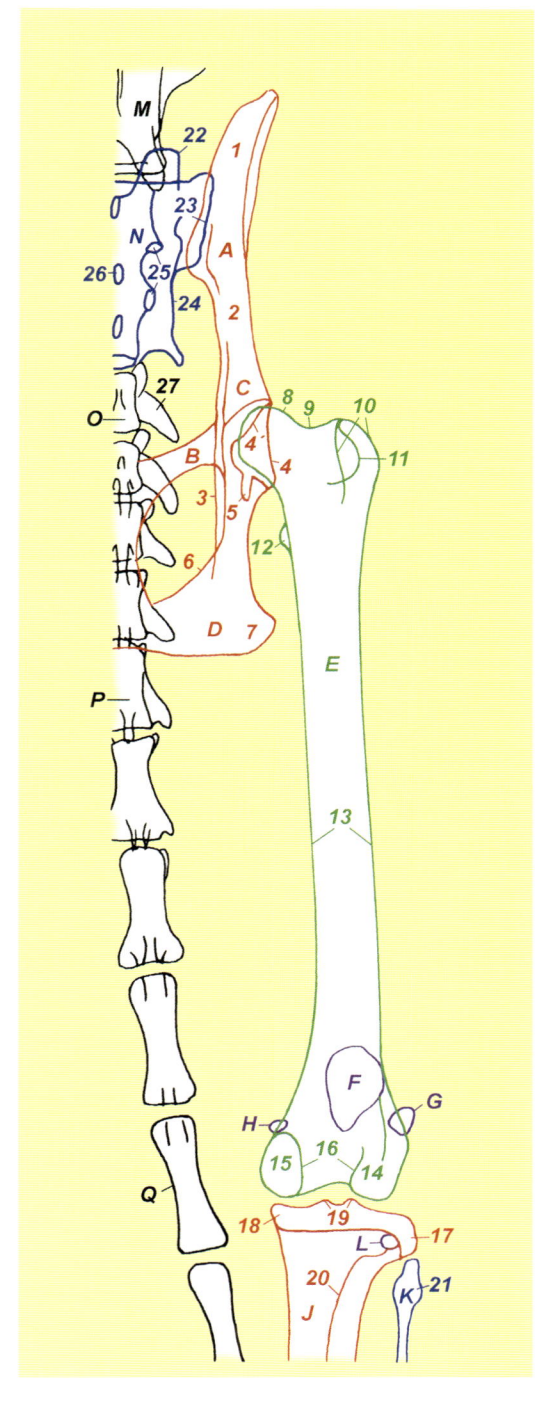

A **Os ilium**
  1   Ala ossis ilii
  2   Corpus ossis ilii

B **Os pubis**

C **Os coxae**
  3   Spina ischiadica
  4   Acetabulum, dorsaler Rand – *dorsal border*
  4' Acetabulum, ventraler Rand – *ventral border*
  5   Incisura acetabuli

D **Os ischii**
  6   Foramen obturatum
  7   Tuber ischiadicum

E **Os femoris**
  8   Caput ossis femoris
  9   Collum ossis femoris
  10 Trochanter major
  11 Fossa trochanterica
  12 Trochanter minor
  13 Corpus ossis femoris
  14 Condylus lateralis
  15 Condylus medialis
  16 Fossa intercondylaris

F **Patella**

G **Os sesamoideum m. gastrocnemii laterale**

H **Os sesamoideum m. gastrocnemii mediale**

J **Tibia**
  17 Condylus lateralis
  18 Condylus medialis
  19 Eminentia intercondylaris
  20 Margo cranialis

K **Fibula**
  21 **Caput fibulae**

L **Os sesamoideum m. poplitei**

M **L VII**

N **Os sacrum**
  22 Processus articularis cranialis
  23 Ala sacralis
  24 Pars lateralis
  25 Foramina sacralia
  26 Processus spinosus

O **Co I**
  27 Processus transversus

P **Co V**

Q **Co IX**

■ **Ziel**
Kranio-kaudale Darstellung des Os femoris mit Hüft- und Kniegelenk.

■ **Zentralstrahl**
Auf die Mitte des Os femoris, die Kassette liegt kaudal dem Oberschenkel an.

■ **Beachte**
Die betroffene Beckengliedmaße liegt auf der Kassette.

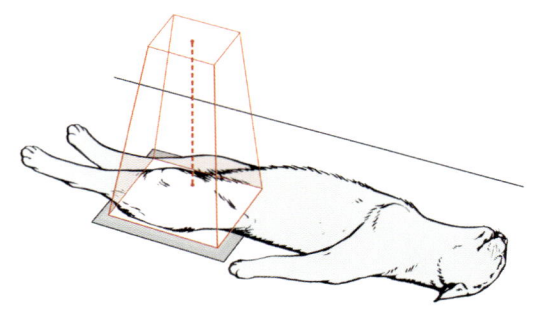

Abb. 4.6 Lagerung zur Aufnahme des Oberschenkels. Kranio-kaudal.

Fig. 4.6 Positioning of the thigh. Cranio-caudal.

■ *Objective*
To obtain a cranio-caudal radiograph of the femur, including the hip and stifle joints.

■ *Central ray of the primary beam*
Place the cassette on the caudal surface of the thigh, direct the x-ray beam perpendicular to the cassette, with the central ray centered in the middle of the femur.

■ *Notice*
The dependent limb lies on the cassette.

4 Beckengliedmaße – Pelvic limb

A Os femoris
  1 Trochlea ossis femoris, lateraler Rollkamm – *lateral ridge*
  2 Trochlea ossis femoris, medialer Rollkamm – *medial ridge*
  3 Trochlea ossis femoris, Furche – *groove*
  4 Condylus lateralis
  5 Condylus medialis
  6 Fossa intercondylaris

B Patella

C Os sesamoideum m. gastrocnemii laterale

D Os sesamoideum m. gastrocnemii mediale

E Tibia
  7 Tuberositas tibiae
  8 Margo cranialis
  9 Condylus lateralis
  10 Condylus medialis
  11 Eminentia intercondylaris
  12 Incisura poplitea

F Fibula
  13 Caput fibulae

G Os sesamoideum m. poplitei

Abb. 4.7 Linkes Kniegelenk, medio-lateral,
Katze
(Ausschnitt aus 13 × 18 cm)

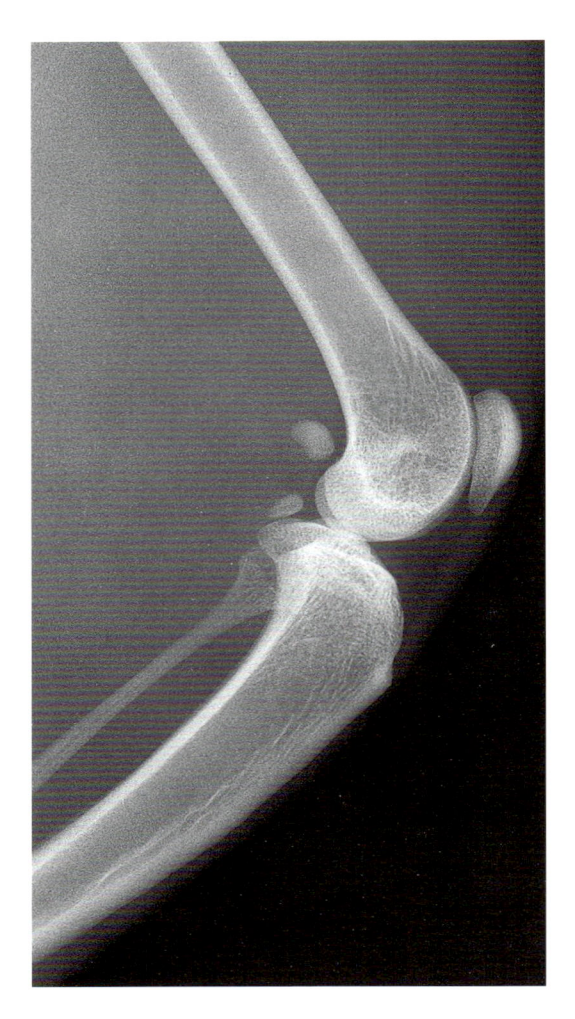

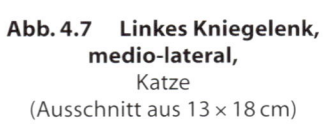

Fig. 4.7 Left stifle joint, medio-lateral,
Cat
(section of 13 × 18 cm)

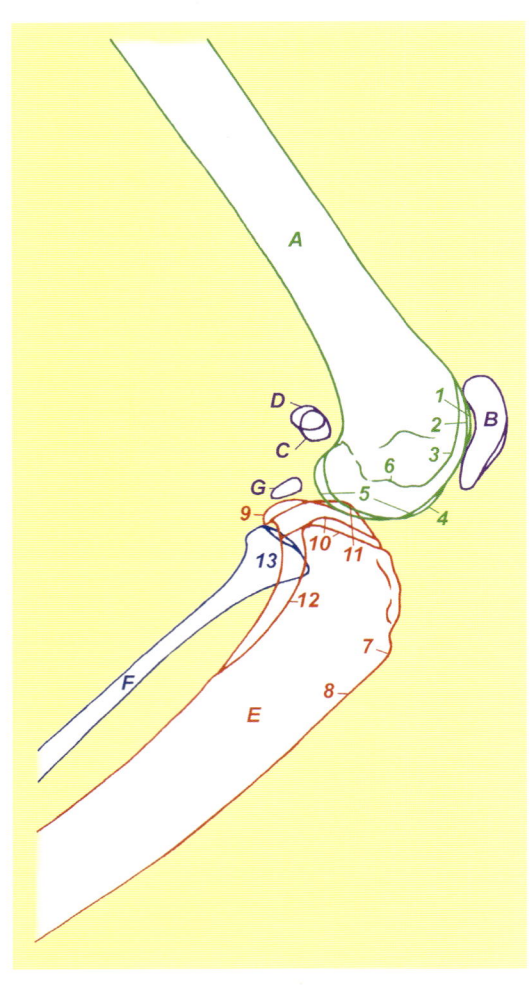

■ **Ziel**
Seitliche Darstellung des Kniegelenks mit den Sesambeinen.

■ **Zentralstrahl**
Auf den Gelenkspalt des Kniekehlgelenks.

■ **Beachte**
Abduktion der oben liegenden Beckengliedmaße.

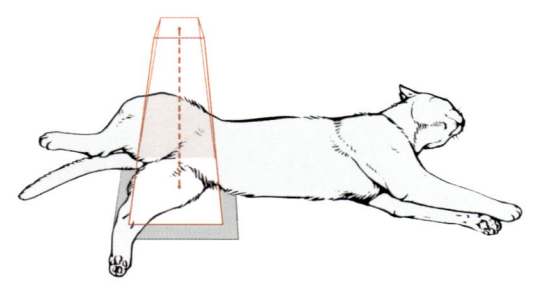

Abb. 4.7 Lagerung zur Aufnahme des Kniegelenks. Medio-lateral.

Fig. 4.7 Positioning of the stifle. Medio-lateral.

■ *Objective*
To obtain a medio-lateral radiograph of the stifle joint, including the sesamoid bones.

■ *Central ray of the primary beam*
Center the central ray of the x-ray beam on the joint space of the stifle.

■ *Notice*
Abduct the nondependent pelvic limb.

4.8 Rechtes Kniegelenk – Right stifle joint ■ kranio-kaudal – cranio-caudal

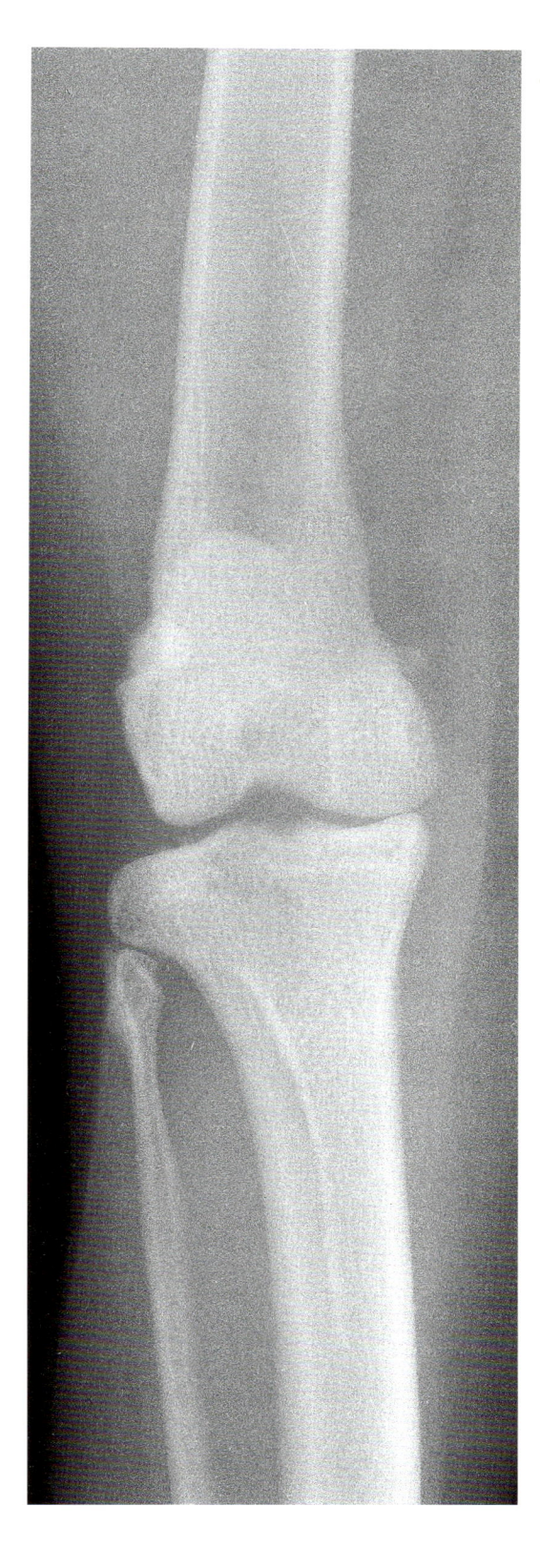

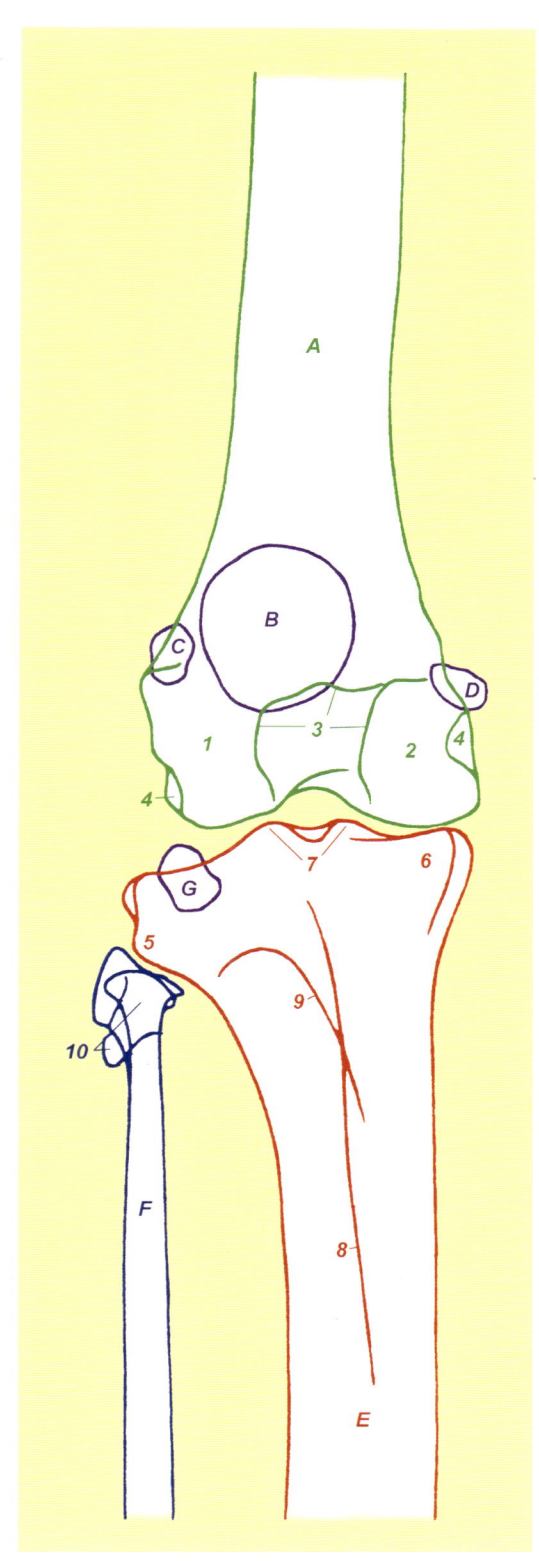

Abb. 4.8 Rechtes Kniegelenk, kranio-kaudal,
Katze
(Ausschnitt aus 13 × 18 cm)

Fig. 4.8 Right stifle joint, cranio-caudal,
Cat
(section of 13 × 18 cm)

A Os femoris
1 Condylus lateralis
2 Condylus medialis
3 Fossa intercondylaris
4 Bandgruben – *depressions for ligamentous attachment*

B Patella

C Os sesamoideum m. gastrocnemii laterale

D Os sesamoideum m. gastrocnemii mediale

E Tibia
5 Condylus lateralis
6 Condylus medialis
7 Eminentia intercondylaris (Tubercula intercondylaria lateralis et medialis)
8 Margo cranialis
9 Incisura poplitea

F Fibula
10 Caput fibulae

G Os sesamoideum m. poplitei

■ **Ziel**
Kranio-kaudale Darstellung des Kniegelenks mit den Sesambeinen.

■ **Zentralstrahl**
Senkrecht zur Kassette, dicht proximal der Tuberositas tibiae.

■ **Beachte**
Beckengliedmaße nach kaudal gestreckt fixiert, leichte Innenrotation der Tibia, Schaumgummikeil unter dem Kniegelenk erleichtert die Lagerung.

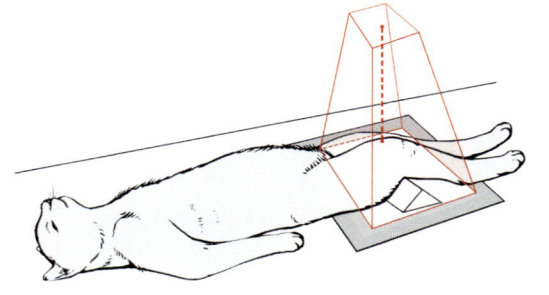

Abb. 4.8 Lagerung zur Aufnahme des Kniegelenks. Kranio-kaudal.

Fig. 4.8 Positioning of the stifle. Cranio-caudal.

■ *Objective*
To obtain a cranio-caudal radiograph of the stifle joint, including the sesamoid bones.

■ *Central ray of the primary beam*
Direct the x-ray beam perpendicular to the cassette, with the central ray centered slightly proximal to the tibial tuberosity.

■ *Notice*
Stretch the pelvic limbs caudally and pronate the tibia slightly, foam rubber wedges supporting the stifle facilitate correct positioning.

4 Beckengliedmaße – Pelvic limb

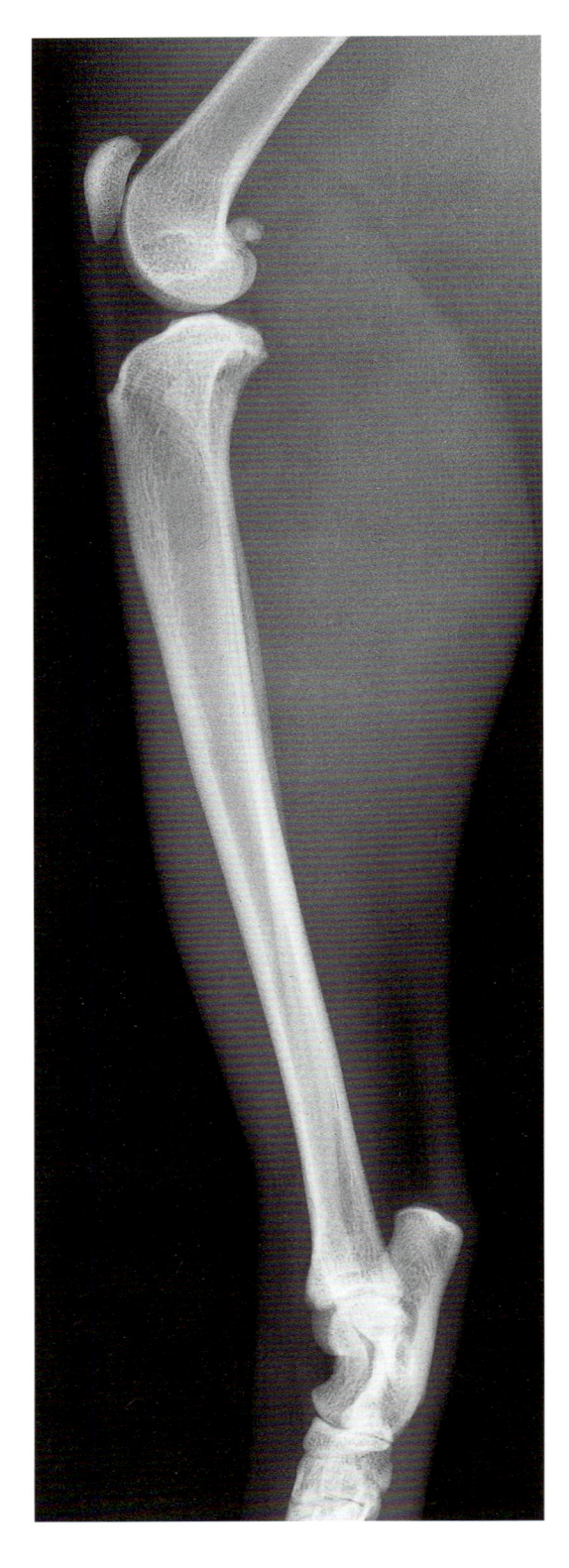

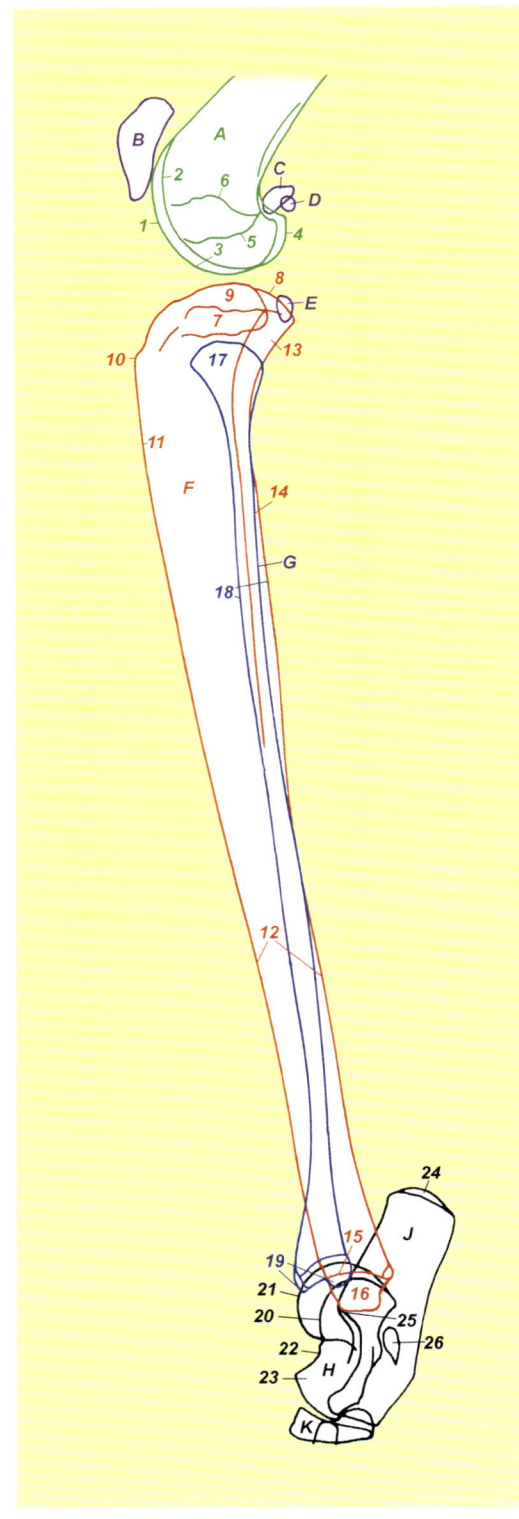

Abb. 4.9 Rechter Unterschenkel, medio-lateral,
Katze
(Ausschnitt aus 18 × 24 cm)

Fig. 4.9 Right lower leg, medio-lateral,
Cat
(section of 18 × 24 cm)

A Os femoris
1 Trochlea ossis femoris, lateraler Rollkamm – *lateral ridge*
2 Trochlea ossis femoris, medialer Rollkamm – *medial ridge*
3 Condylus lateralis
4 Condylus medialis
5 Fossa intercondylaris, Fundus
6 distale Epiphysenfugennarbe – *scar of the distal epiphyseal plate*

B Patella

C Os sesamoideum m. gastrocnemii laterale

D Os sesamoideum m. gastrocnemii mediale

E Os sesamoideum m. poplitei

F Tibia
7 Condylus lateralis
8 Condylus medialis
9 Eminentia intercondylaris
10 Tuberositas tibiae
11 Margo cranialis
12 Corpus tibiae
13 Fossa poplitea
14 Margo medialis
15 Cochlea tibiae
16 Malleolus medialis

G Fibula
17 Caput fibulae
18 Corpus fibulae
19 Malleolus lateralis

H Talus
20 Trochlea tali proximalis, lateraler Kamm – *lateral ridge*
21 Trochlea tali proximalis, medialer Kamm – *medial ridge*
22 Collum tali
23 Caput tali

J Calcaneus
24 Tuber calcanei
25 Processus coracoideus
26 Sustentaculum tali

K Os tarsi centrale

■ **Ziel**
Seitliche Darstellung des Unterschenkels mit Kniegelenk und proximaler Etage des Tarsalgelenks.

■ **Zentralstrahl**
Senkrecht zur Kassette, medial auf die Mitte der Tibia.

■ **Beachte**
Abduktion der oben liegenden Beckengliedmaße.

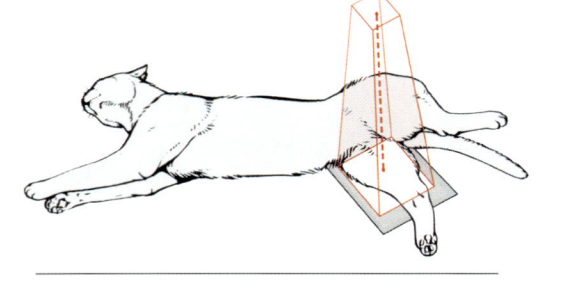

Abb. 4.9 Lagerung zur Aufnahme des Unterschenkels. Medio-lateral.

Fig. 4.9 Positioning of the crus. Medio-lateral.

■ *Objective*
To obtain a medio-lateral radiograph of the lower leg, including stifle joint and the proximal part of the hock joint.

■ *Central ray of the primary beam*
Direct the x-ray beam perpendicular to the cassette, with the central ray centered in the middle of the tibia.

■ *Notice*
Abduct the nondependent pelvic limb.

4.10 Rechter Unterschenkel – Right lower leg ■ kranio-kaudal – cranio-caudal

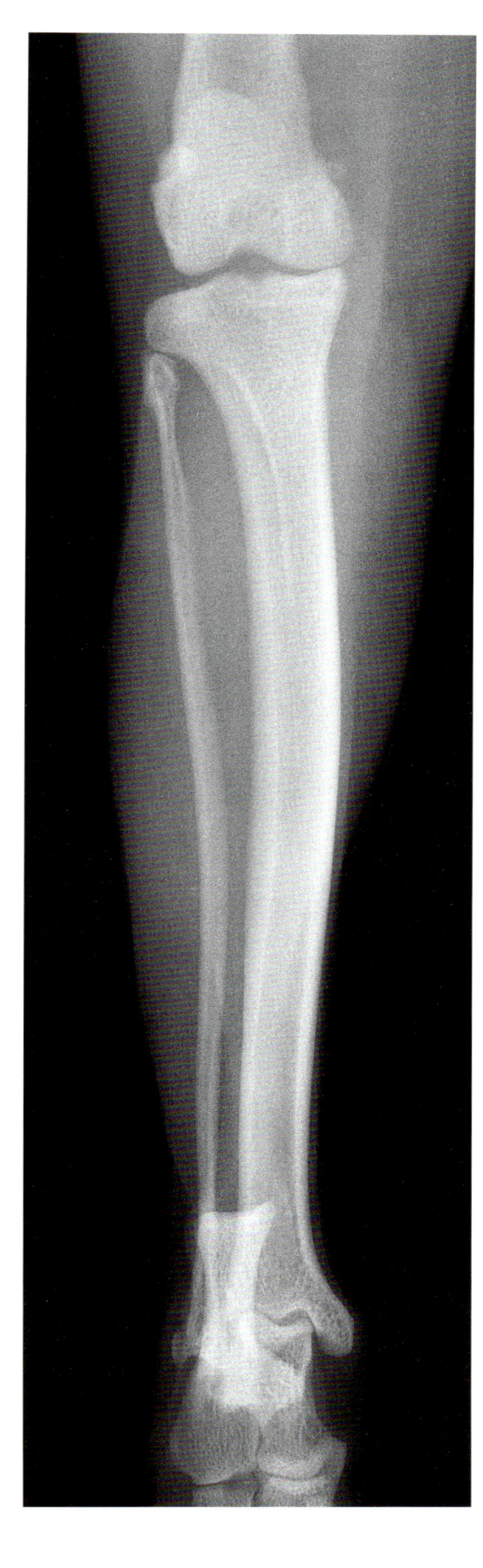

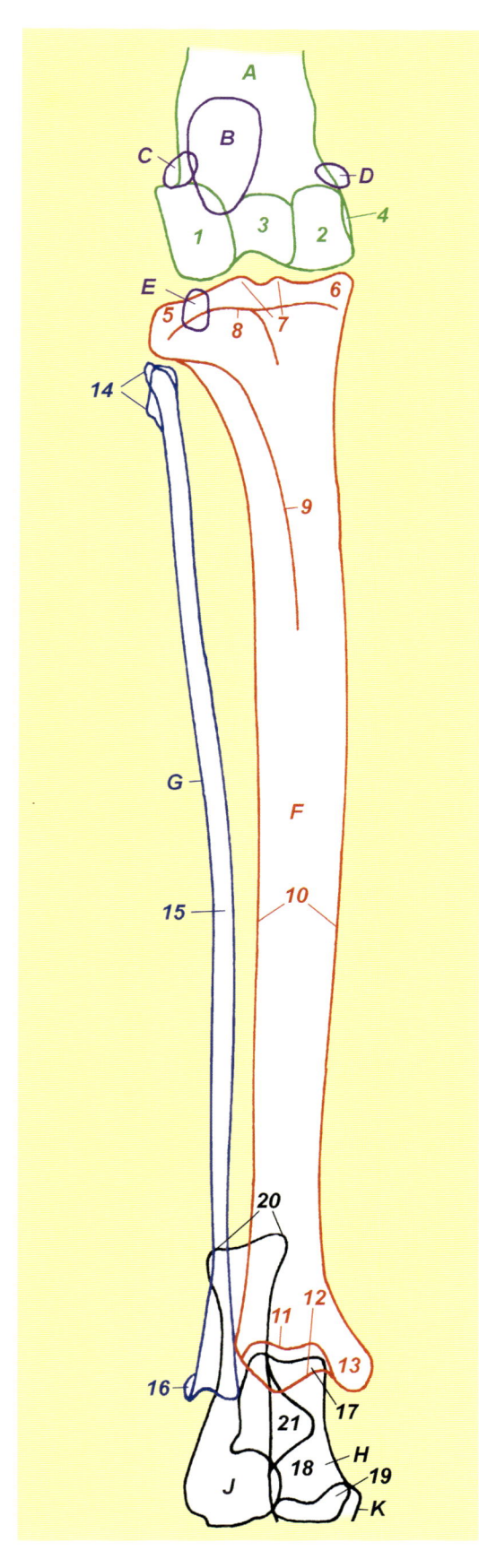

Abb. 4.10 Rechter Unterschenkel, kranio-kaudal,
Katze
(Ausschnitt aus 18 × 24 cm)

Fig. 4.10 Right lower leg, cranio-caudal,
Cat
(section of 18 × 24 cm)

A Os femoris
  1   Condylus lateralis
  2   Condylus medialis
  3   Fossa intercondylaris
  4   Bandgrube – *depression for ligamentous attachment*

B Patella

C Os sesamoideum m. gastrocnemii laterale

D Os sesamoideum m. gastrocnemii mediale

E Os sesamoideum m. poplitei

F Tibia
  5   Condylus lateralis
  6   Condylus medialis
  7   Eminentia intercondylaris
  8   Facies articularis, kaudaler Rand – *caudal border*
  9   Margo cranialis
  10 Corpus tibiae
  11 Cochlea tibiae
  12 Cochlea tibiae, kranialer Rand – *cranial border*
  13 Malleolus medialis

G Fibula
  14 Caput fibulae
  15 Corpus fibulae
  16 Malleolus lateralis

H Talus
  17 Trochlea tali proximalis
  18 Collum tali
  19 Trochlea tali distalis

J Calcaneus
  20 Tuber calcanei
  21 Sustentaculum tali

K Os tarsi centrale

■ **Ziel**
Kranio-kaudale Darstellung des Unterschenkels mit Knie- und proximalem Teil des Tarsalgelenks.

■ **Zentralstrahl**
Senkrecht zur Kassette, kranial auf die Schaftmitte der Tibia.

■ **Beachte**
Die betroffene Beckengliedmaße liegt auf der Kassette, die nicht betroffene Gliedmaße mit dem Schwanz wird abduziert.

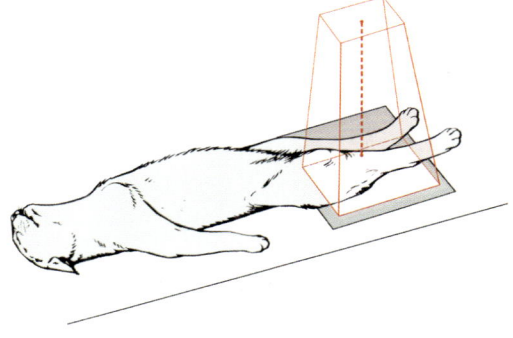

Abb. 4.10 Lagerung zur Aufnahme des Unterschenkels. Kranio-kaudal.

Fig. 4.10 Positioning of the crus. Cranio-caudal.

■ *Objective*
To obtain a cranio-caudal radiograph of the lower leg, including the stifle joint and the proximal part of the hock joint.

■ *Central ray of the primary beam*
Direct the x-ray beam perpendicular to the cassette, with the central ray centered in the middle of the tibia.

■ *Notice*
The patient lies on the cassette, the nondependent pelvic limb is abducted together with the tail.

4 Beckengliedmaße – Pelvic limb

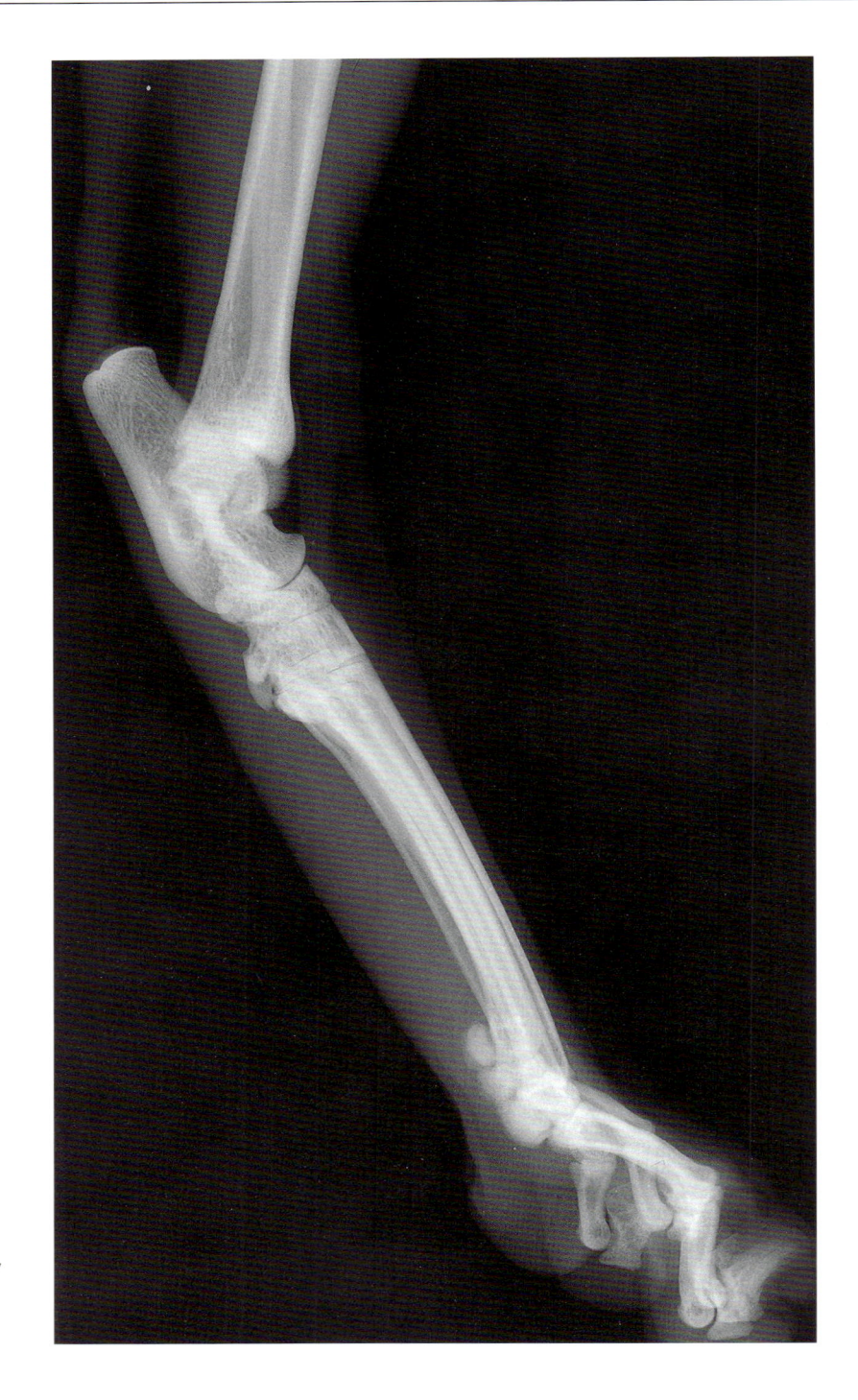

Abb. 4.11 Linker Hinterfuß, medio-lateral,
Katze
(Ausschnitt aus 13 × 18 cm)

Fig. 4.11 Left hindpaw, medio-lateral,
Cat
(section of 13 × 18 cm)

■ **Ziel**
Medio-laterale Darstellung des Hinterfußes mit besonderer Beachtung der Tarsalgelenketagen.

■ **Zentralstrahl**
Senkrecht zur Kassette, auf die Achse des Sprunggelenks in Höhe des Talus.

■ **Beachte**
Der Patient liegt auf der erkrankten Beckengliedmaße, die obere Beckengliedmaße wird kaudal fixiert. Pfote nicht supinieren!

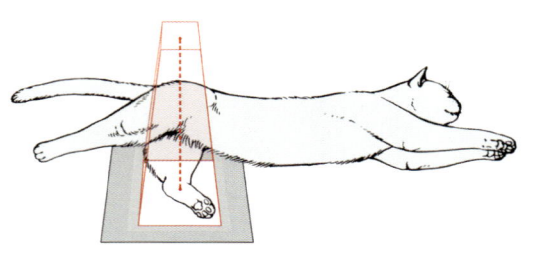

Abb. 4.11 Lagerung zur Aufnahme der Hinterpfote. Medio-lateral.

Fig. 4.11 Positioning of the hindpaw. Medio-lateral.

■ *Objective*
To obtain a medio-lateral radiograph of the hindpaw and adjacent structures of the tibia and fibula.

■ *Central ray of the primary beam*
Direct the x-ray beam perpendicular to the cassette, with the central ray centered in the middle of the talus.

■ *Notice*
Abduct the pelvic limb slightly and stretch it cranially, toes and pads are resting on the supporting surface, do not supinate the hindpaw!

4.11 Linker Hinterfuß – Left hindpaw ■ medio-lateral

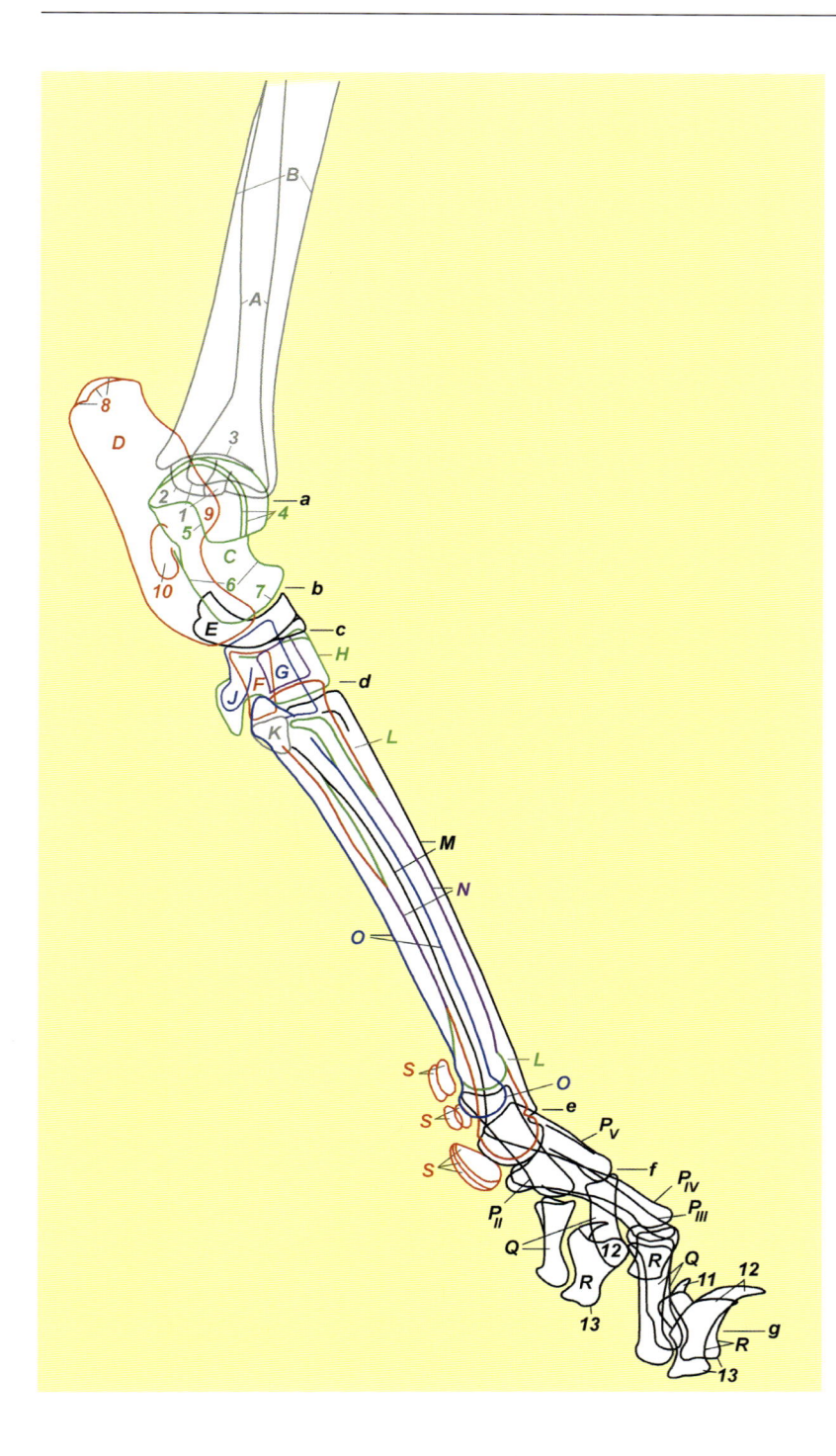

A Fibula
  1 Malleolus lateralis

B Tibia
  2 Malleolus medialis
  3 Cochlea tibiae

C Talus
  4 Trochlea tali proximalis
  5 kaudale Konkavität – *caudal concavity*
  6 Collum tali
  7 Trochlea tali distalis

D Calcaneus
  8 Tuber calcanei
  9 Processus coracoideus
  10 Sustentaculum tali

E Os tarsi centrale

F Os tarsale I

G Os tarsale II

H Os tarsale III

J Os tarsale IV

K Os metatarsale I

L Os metatarsale II

M Os metatarsale III

N Os metatarsale IV

O Os metatarsale V

P Phalanx proximalis

Q Phalanx media

R Phalanx distalis
  11 Crista unguicularis
  12 Processus unguicularis
  13 Tuberositas flexoria

S Ossa sesamoidea proximalia

a Articulatio tarsocruralis

b Articulationes talocalcaneocentralis et calcaneoquartalis

c Articulatio centrodistalis

d Articulationes tarsometatarseae

e Articulatio metatarsophalangea

f Articulatio interphalangea proximalis pedis

g Articulatio interphalangea distalis pedis

4 Beckengliedmaße – Pelvic limb

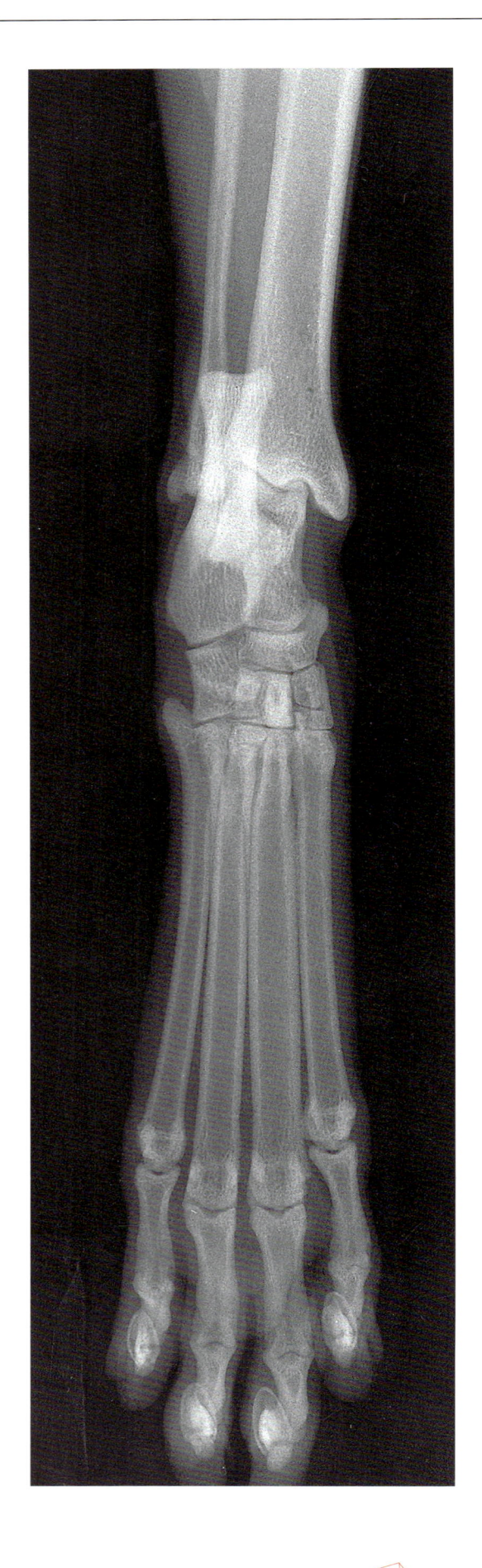

Abb. 4.12 Rechter Hinterfuß, dorso-plantar,
Katze
(Ausschnitt aus 13 x 18 cm)

Fig. 4.12 Right hindpaw, dorso-plantar,
Cat
(section of 13 x 18 cm)

■ **Ziel**
Dorso-plantare Darstellung des Hinterfußes sowie der gelenknahen Abschnitte von Tibia und Fibula.

■ **Zentralstrahl**
Senkrecht zur Kassette, dorsal auf die Mitte des Talus.

■ **Beachte**
Beckengliedmaße in leichter Abduktion kaudal gestreckt, Zehen und Sohlenballen liegen der Unterlage an.

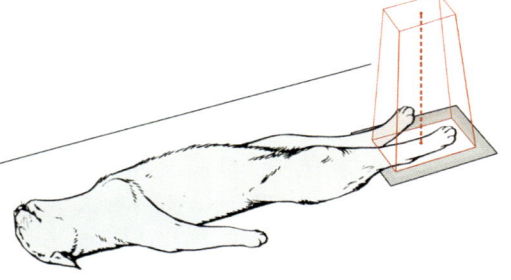

Abb. 4.12 Lagerung zur Aufnahme der Hinterpfote. Dorso-plantar.

Fig. 4.12 Positioning of the hindpaw. Dorso-plantar.

■ **Objective**
To obtain a dorso-plantar radiograph of the hindpaw and adjacent structures of the tibia and fibula.

■ **Central ray of the primary beam**
Direct the x-ray beam perpendicular to the cassette, with the central ray centered in the middle of the talus.

■ **Notice**
Abduct the pelvic limb slightly and stretch it caudally, toes and pads are resting on the supporting surface.

4.12 Rechter Hinderfuß – Right hindpaw ■ dorso-plantar

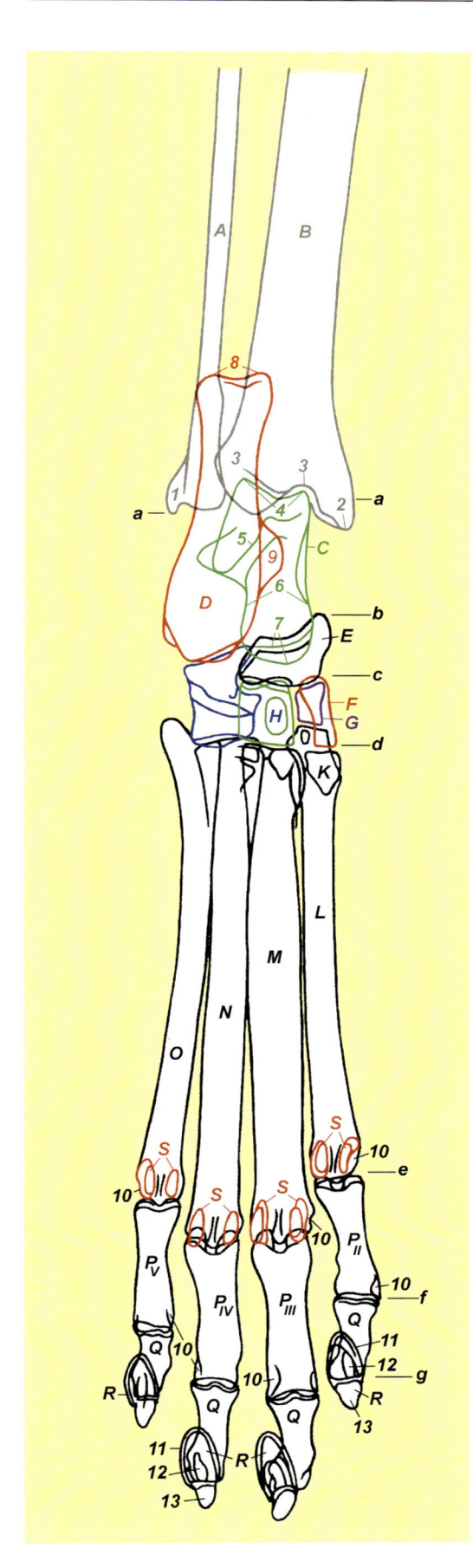

A **Fibula**
  1   Malleolus lateralis

B **Tibia**
  2   Malleolus medialis
  3   Cochlea tibiae

C **Talus**
  4   Trochlea tali proximalis
  5   Sulcus tali
  6   Collum tali
  7   Trochlea tali distalis

D **Calcaneus**
  8   Tuber calcanei
  9   Sustentaculum tali

E **Os tarsi centrale**

F **Os tarsale I**

G **Os tarsale II**

H **Os tarsale III**

J **Os tarsale IV**

K **Os metatarsale I**

L **Os metatarsale II**

M **Os metatarsale III**

N **Os metatarsale IV**

O **Os metatarsale V**
  10 Bandgruben – *depressions for ligamentous attachment*

P **Phalanx proximalis**

Q **Phalanx media**

R **Phalanx distalis**
  11 Crista unguicularis
  12 Processus unguicularis
  13 Tuberositas flexoria

S **Ossa sesamoidea proximalia**

a **Articulatio tarsocruralis**

b **Articulationes talocalcaneocentralis et calcaneoquartalis**

c **Articulatio centrodistalis**

d **Articulationes tarsometatarseae**

e **Articulatio metatarsophalangea**

f **Articulatio interphalangea proximalis pedis**

g **Articulatio interphalangea distalis pedis**

4 Beckengliedmaße – Pelvic limb

Tabelle 4.1 Zeitliches Auftreten der Ossifikationspunkte sowie des Apo- und Epiphysenfugenschlusses am Skelett der Beckengliedmaße der Hauskatze (nach A. HORVATH, 1983)

Table 4.1 Time-table of the appearance of ossification centers and closures of apo- and epiphyseal lines of the pelvic limb in the domestic cat (after A. HORVATH, 1983)

Ossifikationspunkte Apo- und Epiphysen *Ossification centers Apophyses and Epiphyses*	Auftreten der Ossifikationspunkte (Angabe in Tagen) *Appearance of the ossification centers (in days)*	Apo- und Epiphysenfugenschluss (Angabe in Monaten) *Fusion of epi- and apophyseal lines (in months)*
OS COXAE		
Os ilium	prenatal	8–9*
Os ischii	prenatal	8–9*
Os pubis	prenatal	8–9*
Os acetabuli	62–69	8–9*
Crista iliaca	183–231	>26
Tuberculum ischiadicum	58–73	>26
OS FEMORIS		
Epiphysis proximalis (Caput)	13–17	11–12
Trochanter major	20–24	11–14
Trochanter minor	13–17	12–15
Epiphysis distalis ossis femoris	13–17	17–20
TIBIA		
Epiphysis proximalis tibiae	14–21	17–21
Tuberositas tibiae	48–59	17–22
Epiphysis distalis tibiae	15–24	12–14
FIBULA		
Epiphysis proximalis fibulae	36–58	17–21
Epiphysis distalis fibulae	22–31	12–14
OSSA TARSI		
Tuber calcanei (Apophysis)	34–45	11–15*
Os tarsi centrale	28–42	
Os tarsale I	29–43	
Os tarsale II	35–43	
Os tarsale III	29–42	
Os tarsale IV	28–42	
OSSA METATARSALIA		
Os metatarsale I	58–113	
Epiphysis distalis		
– ossium metatarsalium II, V	28–31	10–12
– ossium metatarsalium III, IV	27–31	10–12
OSSA DIGITORUM PEDIS		
Epiphysis proximalis		
– phalangium proximalium II, V	28–36	7–9
– phalangium proximalium III, IV	22–31	7–9
– phalangium mediarum II, V	28–35	6–8
– phalangium mediarum III, IV	24–29	6–8
OSSA SESAMOIDEA		
Patella	56–100	
Os sesamoideum laterale m. gastrocnemii	84–142	
Os sesamoideum mediale m. gastrocnemii	154–239	
Os sesamoideum m. poplitei	141–183	
Os sesamoideum proximalia digitorum II, V	84–127	
Os sesamoideum proximalia digitorum III, IV	84–113	

* Fusion von Ossifikationskernen – *fusion of ossification centers*

4 Beckengliedmaße – Pelvic limb

d 24   d 45   d 102   d 157   d 255   d 297   d 366   d 404   d 499

Abb. 4.13 Postnatale Entwicklung,
linke Beckenhälfte und linkes Hüftgelenk,
ventro-dorsal,
Katze,
Lebensalter in Tagen (d)

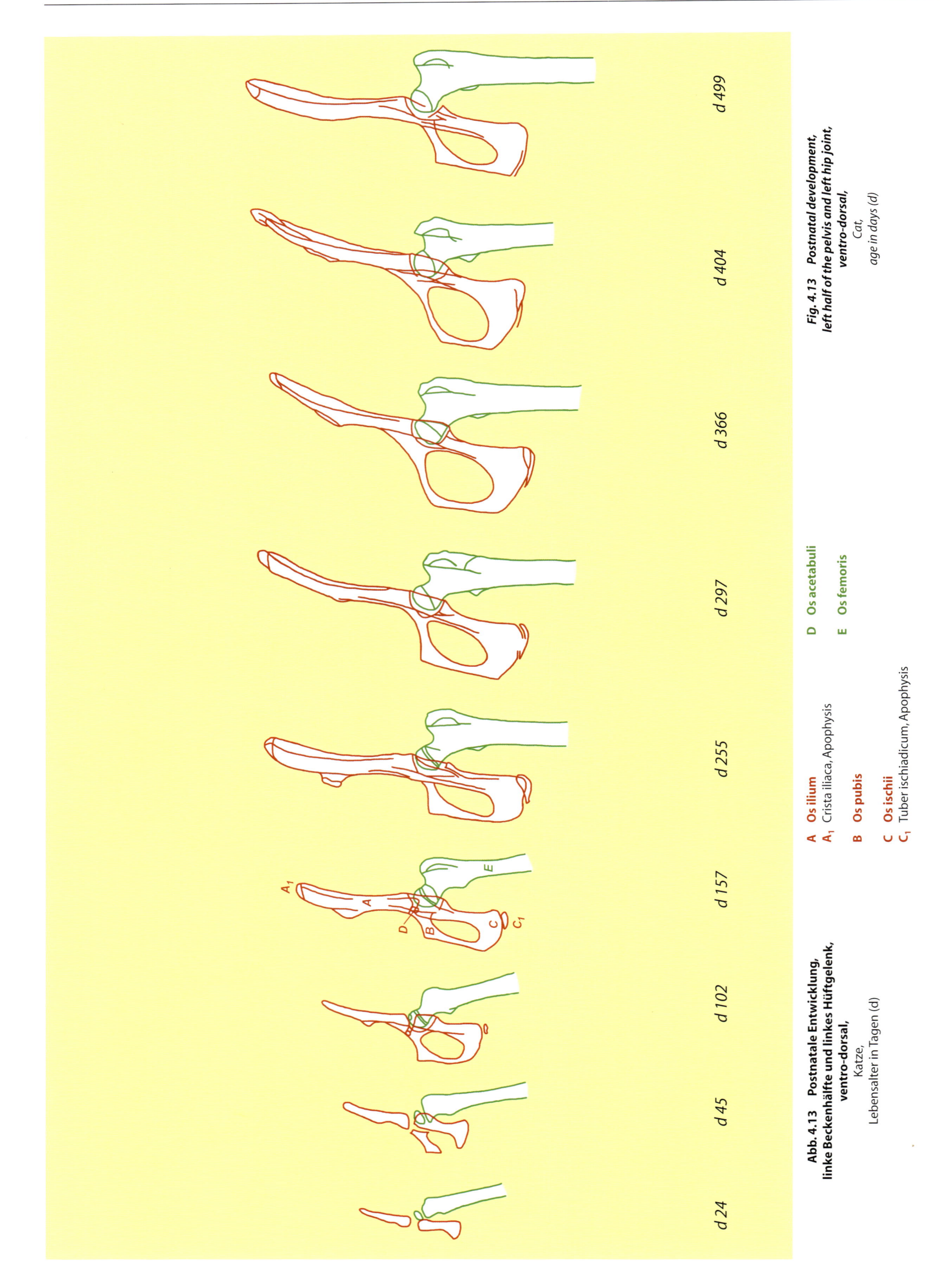

A   Os ilium
A₁ Crista iliaca, Apophysis
B   Os pubis
C   Os ischii
C₁ Tuber ischiadicum, Apophysis

D   Os acetabuli
E   Os femoris

Fig. 4.13 Postnatal development,
left half of the pelvis and left hip joint,
ventro-dorsal,
Cat,
age in days (d)

4.14/4.15 Postnatale Entwicklung – Postnatal development ■ Kniegelenk – stifle joint

Abb. 4.14 Postnatale Entwicklung linkes Kniegelenk, medio-lateral,
Katze, Lebensalter in Tagen (d)

Abb. 4.15 Postnatale Entwicklung, rechtes Kniegelenk, kranio-kaudal,
Katze, Lebensalter in Tagen (d)

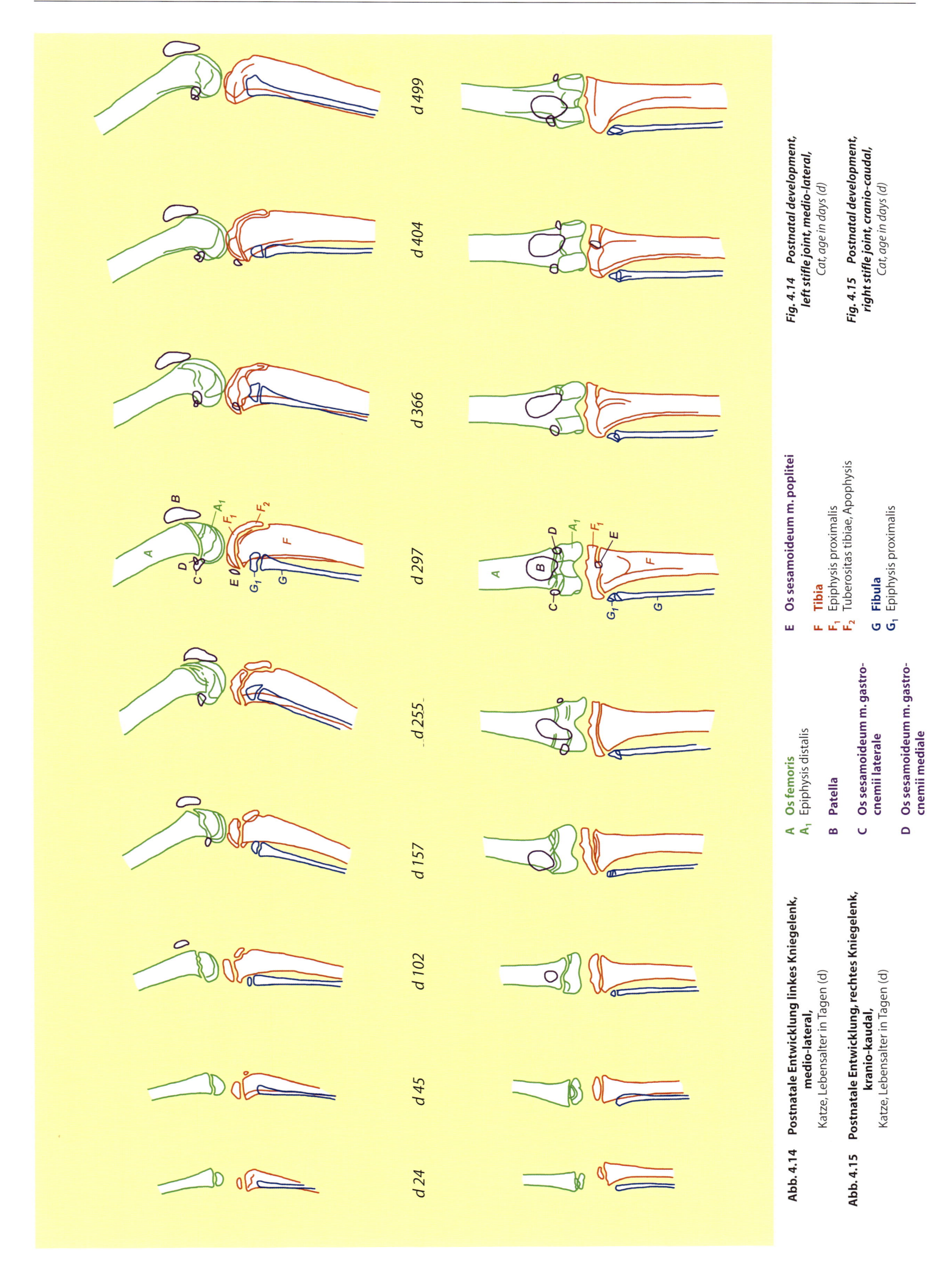

Fig. 4.14 Postnatal development, left stifle joint, medio-lateral,
Cat, age in days (d)

Fig. 4.15 Postnatal development, right stifle joint, cranio-caudal,
Cat, age in days (d)

A **Os femoris**
A_1 Epiphysis distalis
B **Patella**
C Os sesamoideum m. gastrocnemii laterale
D Os sesamoideum m. gastrocnemii mediale
E Os sesamoideum m. poplitei
F **Tibia**
F_1 Epiphysis proximalis
F_2 Tuberositas tibiae, Apophysis
G **Fibula**
G_1 Epiphysis proximalis

d 24, d 45, d 102, d 157, d 255, d 297, d 366, d 404, d 499

79

4 Beckengliedmaße – Pelvic limb

Abb. 4.16 Postnatale Entwicklung, linkes Tarsalgelenk, medio-lateral, Katze, Lebensalter in Tagen (d)

Abb. 4.17 Postnatale Entwicklung, rechter Hinterfuß, dorso-plantar, Katze, Lebensalter in Tagen (d)

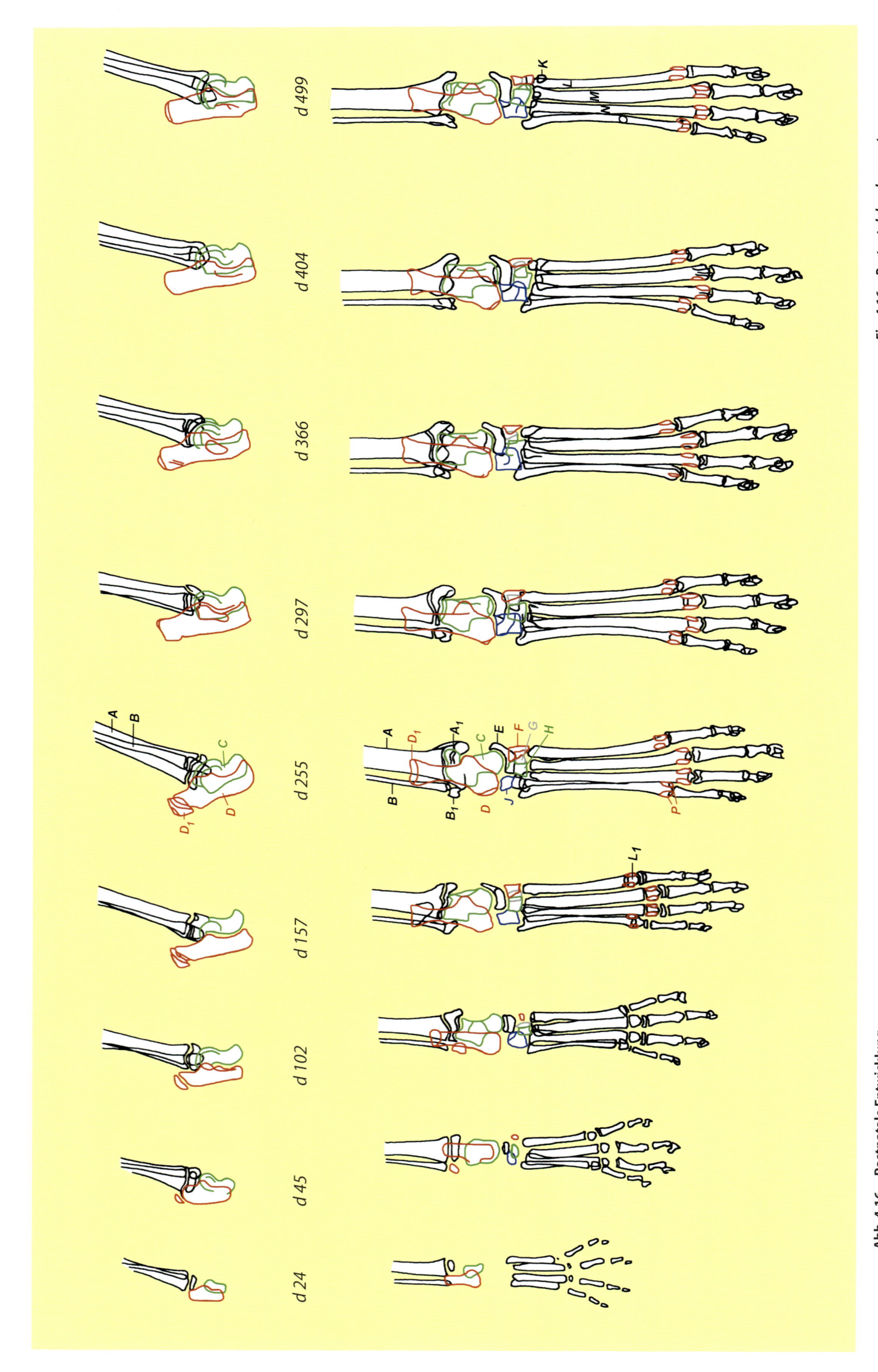

Fig. 4.16 Postnatal development, left hock joint, medio-lateral, Cat, age in days (d)

Fig. 4.17 Postnatal development, right hindpaw, dorso-plantar, Cat, age in days (d)

80

A Tibia	**E Os tarsi centrale**	**L Os metatarsale II**
A₁ Cochlea tibiae, Epiphysis distalis	**F Os tarsale I**	L₁ Epiphysis (distal)
B Fibula	**G Os tarsale II**	**M Os metatarsale III**
B₁ Malleolus lateralis, Epiphysis distalis	**H Os tarsale III**	**N Os metatarsale IV**
C Talus	**J Os tarsale IV**	**O Os metatarsale V**
D Calcaneus	**K Os metatarsale I**	**P Ossa sesamoidea proximalia**
D₁ Tuber calcanei, Apophysis		

5 Thorax – Thorax

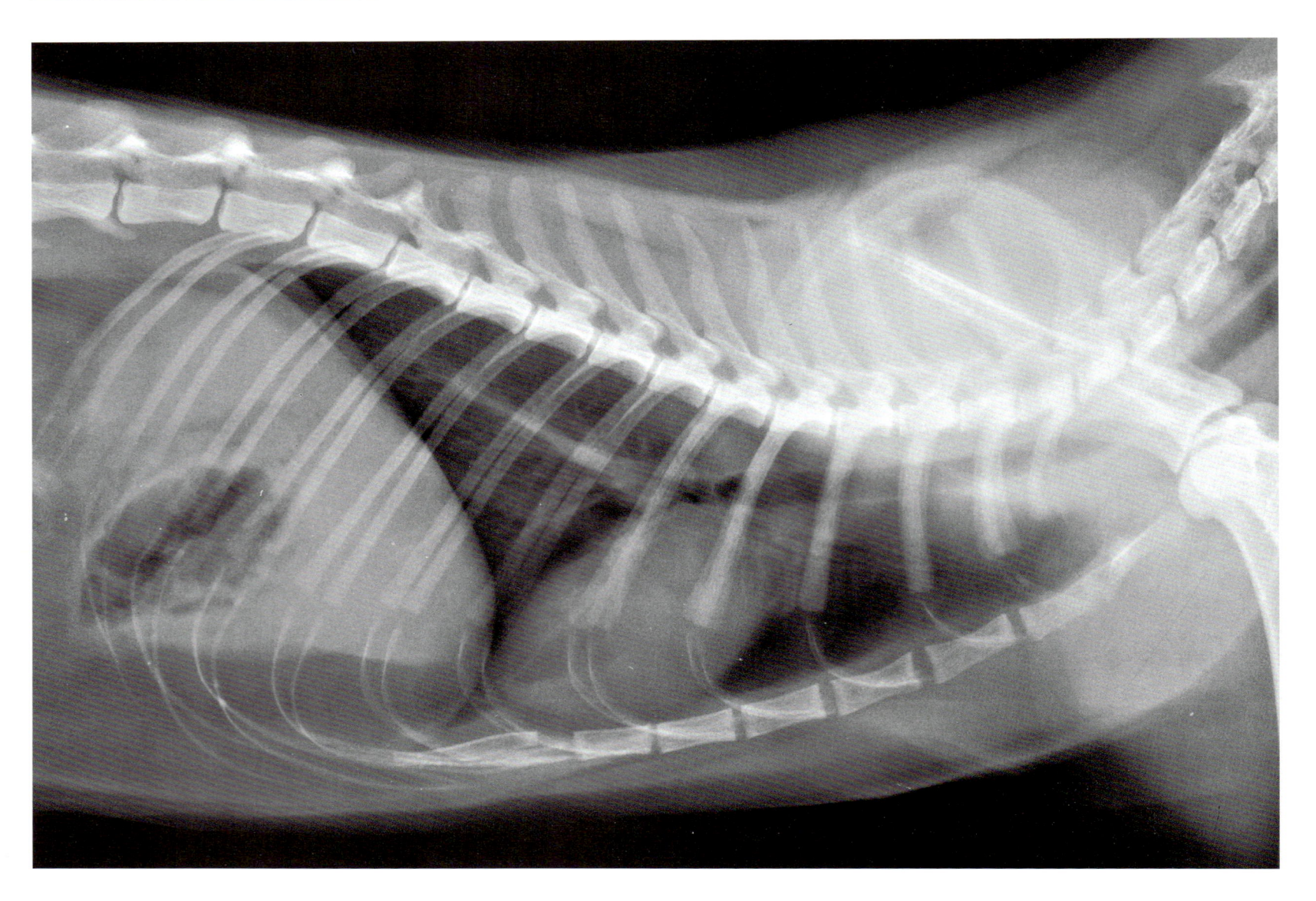

Abb. 5.1 Thorax, liegend, latero-lateral,
Katze
(Ausschnitt aus 24 × 30 cm)

Fig. 5.1 Thorax, recumbent, latero-lateral,
Cat
(section of 24 × 30 cm)

■ **Ziel**
Darstellung der Brustorgane.

■ **Zentralstrahl**
Senkrecht zur Kassette, in halber Höhe des 7. Brustwirbels.

■ **Beachte**
Streckung der Schultergliedmaßen nach vorn und der Beckengliedmaßen nach hinten.

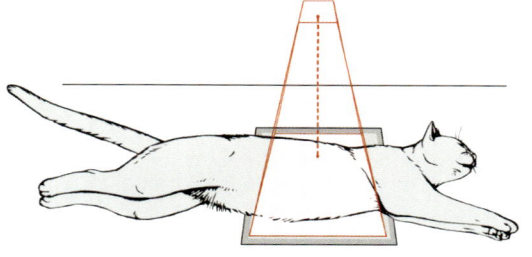

Abb. 5.1 Lagerung zur Aufnahme des Thorax. Latero-lateral.

Fig. 5.1 Positioning of the thorax. Latero-lateral.

■ *Objective*
To image the thoracic organs.

■ *Central ray of the primary beam*
Direct the x-ray beam perpendicular to the cassette, with the central ray centered at the level of T 7.

■ *Notice*
Stretch the thoracic limbs cranially and the pelvic limbs caudally.

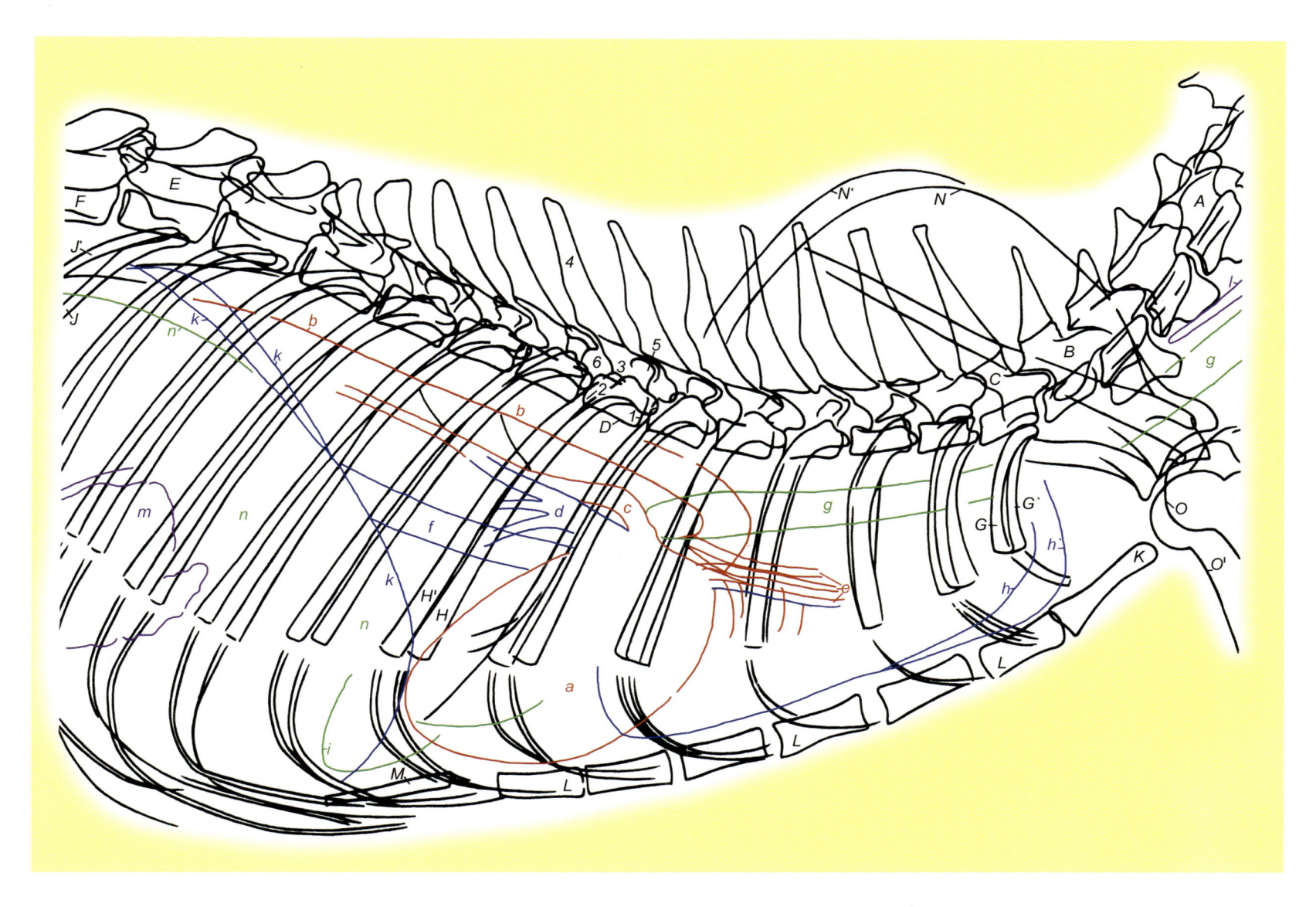

5.1 Thorax – Thorax ■ latero-lateral

A C IV	H Os costale VII, H´ plattenfern – *next to the tube*	d Vv. pulmonales
B C VII		e **Aa. pulmonales mit Vena cava cranialis** (Ventralrand – v*entral border*)
C T I	J Os costale XIII, J´ plattenfern – *next to the tube*	
D T VII		f Vena cava caudalis
1 Facies terminalis cranialis	K Manubrium sterni	g Trachea
2 Facies terminalis caudalis	L Sternebrae	h Cupula pleurae, h´ plattenfern – *next to the tube*
3 Foramen vertebrale	M Processus xiphoideus	
4 Processus spinosus	N Scapula, N´ plattenfern – *next to the tube*	i Lobus medius pulmonis dextri
5 Processus articularis cranialis	O Humerus, O´ plattenfern – *next to the tube*	k Diaphragma
6 Foramen intervertebrale	a Cor	l Oesophagus (Pars cervicalis)
E T XIII	b Aorta thoracica	m Ventriculus
F L I	c Aa. pulmonales	n Hepar
G Os costale I, G´ plattenfern – *next to the tube*		

5 Thorax – Thorax

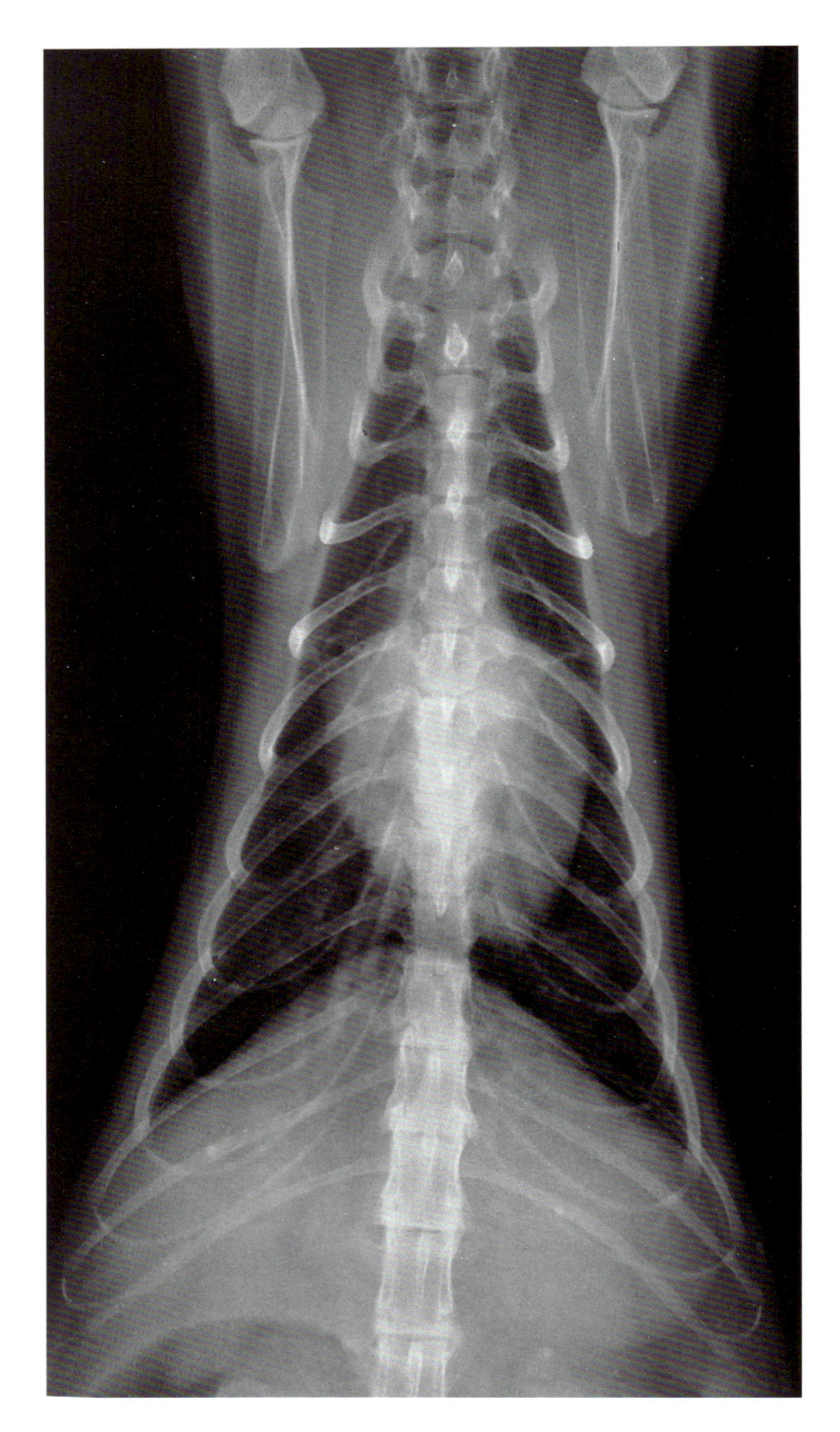

Abb. 5.2 Thorax, ventro-dorsal,
Katze
(Ausschnitt aus 24 × 30 cm)

Fig. 5.2 Thorax, ventro-dorsal,
Cat
(section of 24 × 30 cm)

■ **Ziel**
Darstellung der Brustorgane.

■ **Zentralstrahl**
Senkrecht auf das Brustbein, in Höhe des 7. Brustwirbels.

■ **Beachte**
Symmetrische Streckung der Schultergliedmaßen nach vorn und der Beckengliedmaßen nach hinten; Rückenlage durch Schaumgummikeile seitlich stabilisieren.
Seitenbezeichnung nicht vergessen!

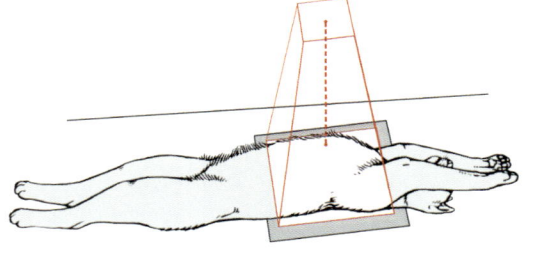

Abb. 5.2 Lagerung zur Aufnahme des Thorax. Ventro-dorsal.

Fig. 5.2 Positioning of the thorax. Ventro-dorsal.

■ *Objective*
To image the thoracic organs.

■ *Central ray of the primary beam*
Direct the x-ray beam perpendicular to the sternum, with the central ray centered at the level of T7.

■ *Notice*
Extend the thoracic limbs cranially and the pelvic limbs caudally, use positioning wedges to support a symmetric dorsal recumbency.
Do not forget the R/L mark!

5.2 Thorax – Thorax ■ ventro-dorsal

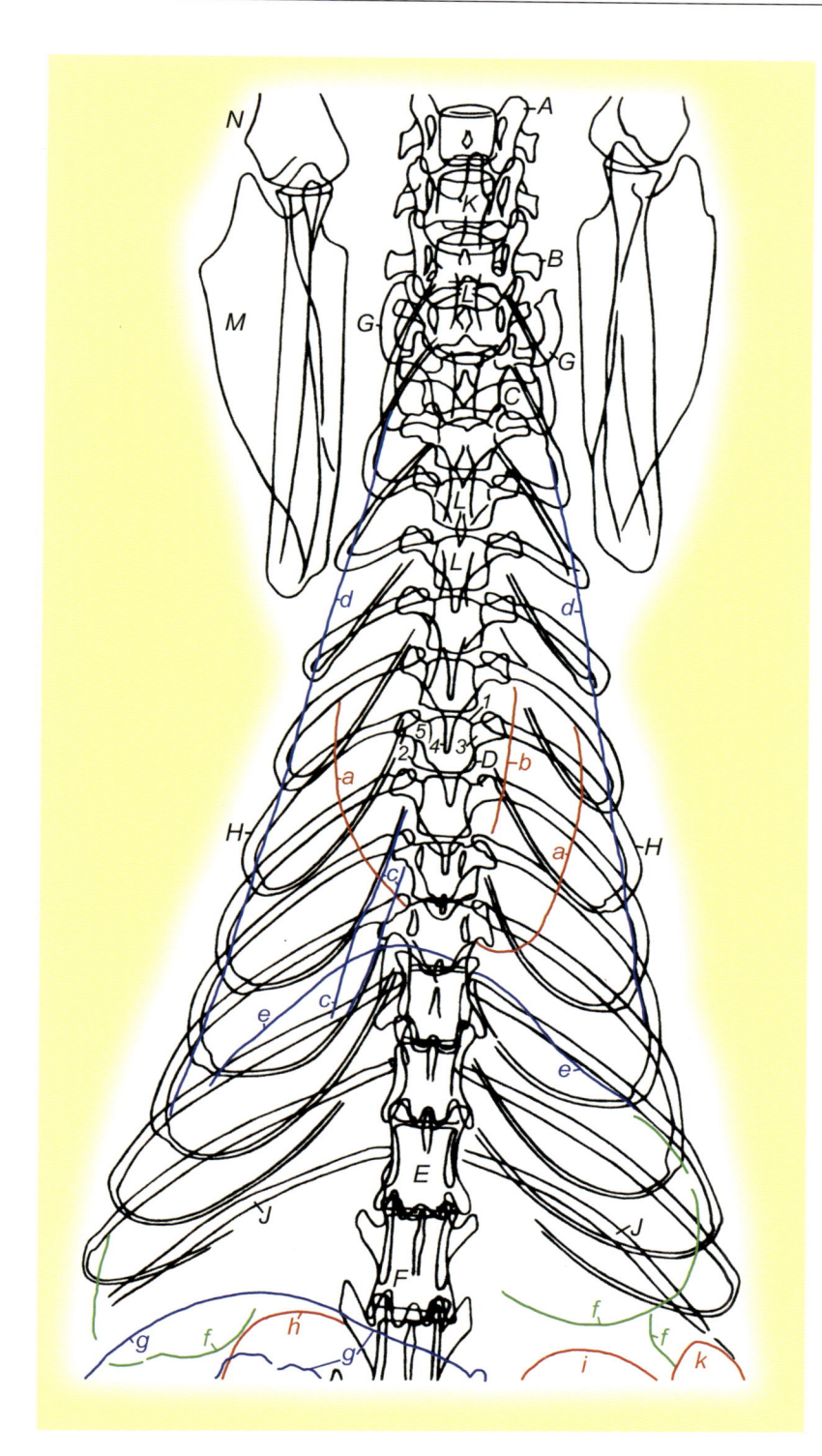

A C IV

B C VI

C T I

D T VII
    1 Facies terminalis cranialis
    2 Facies terminalis caudalis
    3 Pediculus arcus vertebrae
    4 Processus spinosus
    5 Processus transversus

E T XIII

F L I

G Os costale I

H Os costale VII

J Os costale XIII

K Manubrium sterni

L Sternebrae

M Scapula

N Humerus

a Cor

b Aorta thoracica

c Vena cava caudalis

d Cavum pleurae, laterale Wand – *lateral wall*

e Diaphragma

f Hepar

g Intestinum (zum Teil gashaltig – *partly filled with gas*)

h Ren dexter

i Ren sinister

k Lien

5 Thorax – Thorax

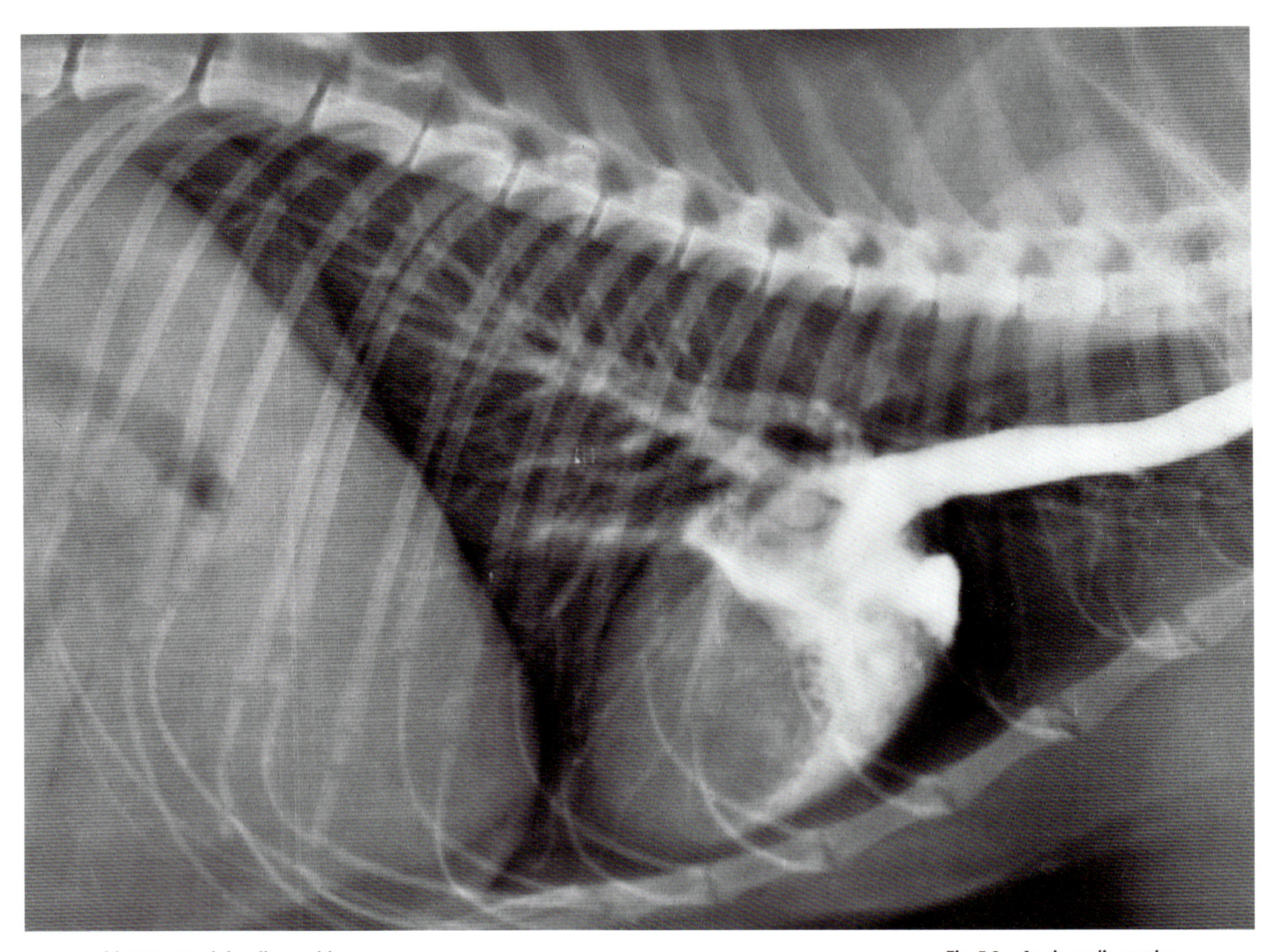

**Abb. 5.3 Angiokardiographie,
Aufnahme aus Bildserie,**
aufgenommen mit Angio-Kardio-
Seriograph nach BUCHTALA
(Urografin 76%, Schering),
Injektion in die V. jugularis externa,
venöse Seite, Endphase der Systole, **liegend,
latero-lateral,**
Katze
(Ausschnitt aus 24 × 30 cm)

*Fig. 5.3 Angiocardiography,
Radiograph out of series,*
*taken by angio-cardio-
seriograph after BUCHTALA
(Urografin 76%, Schering),
injection into external jugular vein,
venous side, end
phase of systole,* **recumbent,
latero-lateral,**
*Cat
(section of 24 × 30 cm)*

■ **Ziel**
Darstellung der Brustorgane.

■ **Zentralstrahl**
Senkrecht zur Kassette, in halber Höhe des 8. Brustwirbels.

■ **Beachte**
Streckung der Schultergliedmaßen nach vorn und der Beckengliedmaßen nach hinten.

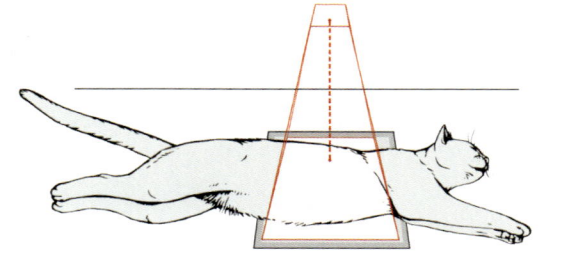

Abb. 5.3 Lagerung zur Aufnahme des Thorax. Latero-lateral.

Fig. 5.3 Positioning of the thorax. Latero-lateral.

■ *Objective*
To image the thoracic organs.

■ *Central ray of the primary beam*
Direct the x-ray beam perpendicular to the cassette, with the central ray centered at the level of T8.

■ *Notice*
Stretch the thoracic limbs cranially and the pelvic limbs caudally.

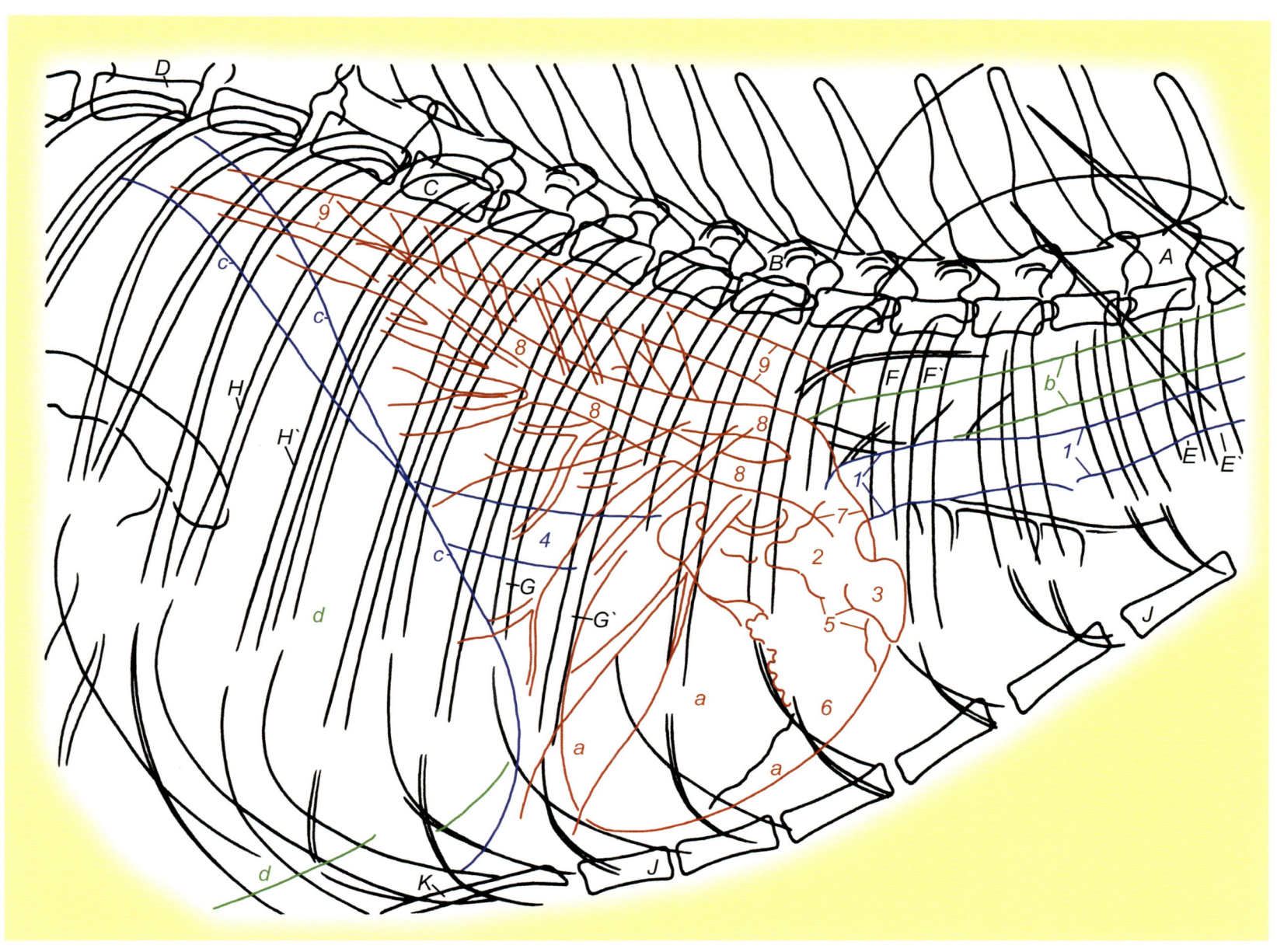

5.3 Angiokardiographie – Angiocardiography ■ latero-lateral

A T I	**G** Os costale VII, G´ plattenfern – *next to the tube*	**4** Vena cava caudalis
B T VI		**5** Ostium atrioventriculare dextrum
C T X	**H** Os costale X, H´ plattenfern – *next to the tube*	**6** Ventriculus dexter
D T XIII		**7** Truncus pulmonalis
	J Sternebrae	**8** Aa. pulmonales
E Os costale I, E´ plattenfern – *next to the tube*	**K** Processus xiphoideus	**9** Aorta thoracica
F Os costale IV, F´ plattenfern – *next to the tube*	**a** Cor	**b Trachea**
	1 Vena cava cranialis	**c Diaphragma**
	2 Atrium dextrum	**d Hepar**
	3 Auricula dextra	

5 Thorax – Thorax

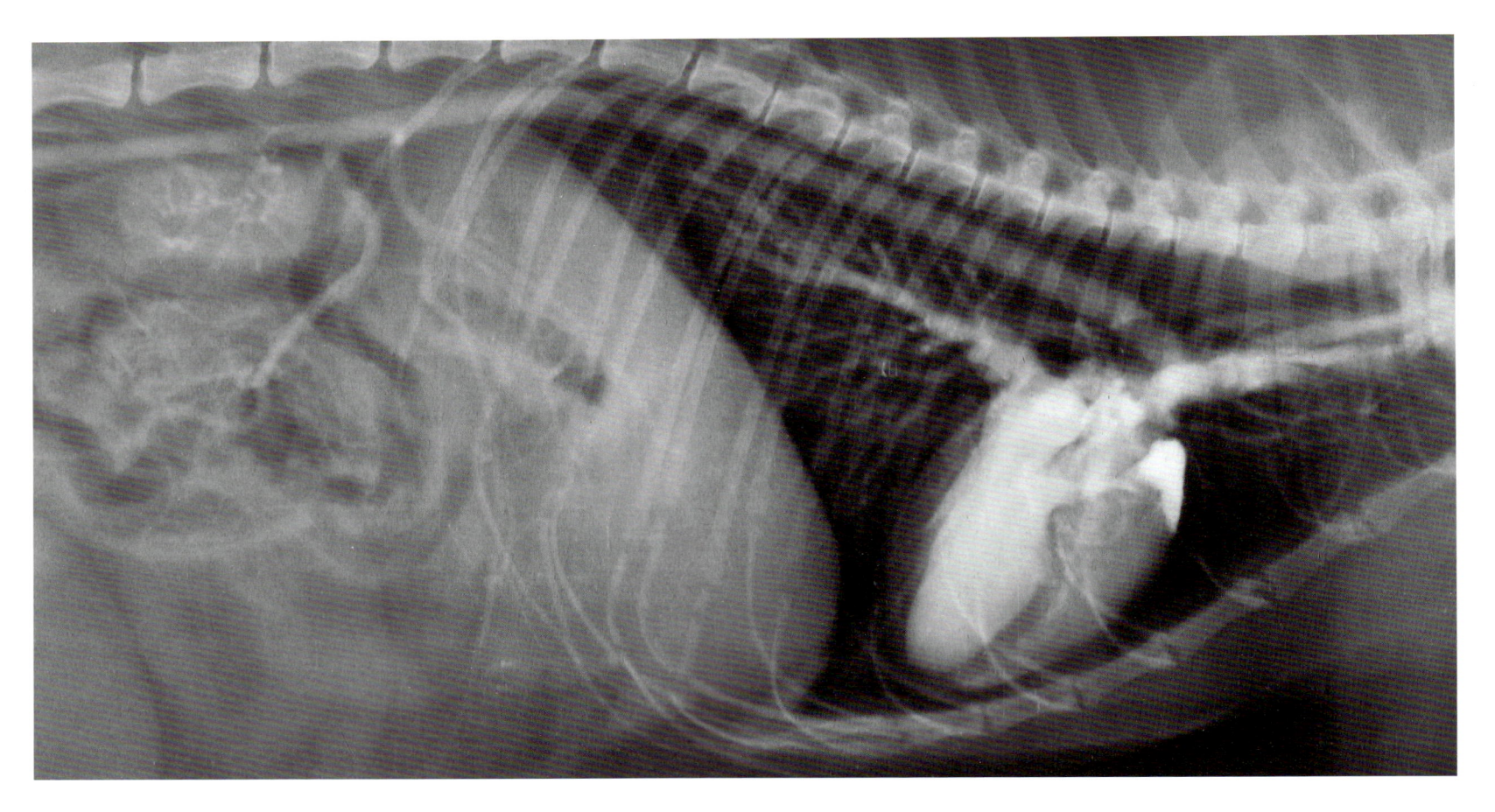

**Abb. 5.4 Angiokardiographie,
Aufnahme aus Bildserie,** aufgenommen
mit Angio-Kardio-Seriograph nach
BUCHTALA (Urografin 76 %, Schering),
Injektion in die V. jugularis externa,
arterielle Seite, Diastole, **liegend,
latero-lateral,**
Katze
(Ausschnitt aus 24 × 30 cm)

*Fig. 5.4 Angiocardiography,
Radiograph out of series, taken by
angio-cardio-seriograph after BUCHTALA
(Urografin 76%, Schering),
injection into external jugular vein,
arterial side, diastole, **recumbent,
latero-lateral,**
Cat
(section of 24 × 30 cm)*

■ **Ziel**
Darstellung der Brustorgane.

■ **Zentralstrahl**
Senkrecht zur Kassette, in halber Höhe des
10. Brustwirbels.

■ **Beachte**
Streckung der Schultergliedmaßen nach
vorn und der Beckengliedmaßen nach
hinten.

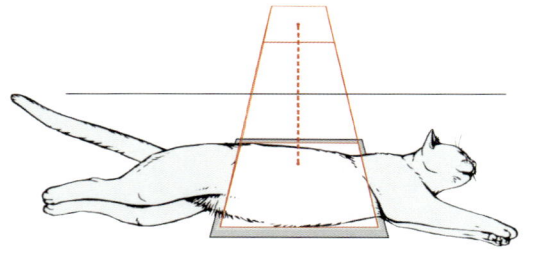

**Abb. 5.4 Lagerung zur Aufnahme des Thorax.
Latero-lateral.**

*Fig. 5.4 Positioning of the thorax.
Latero-lateral.*

■ *Objective*
To image the thoracic organs.

■ *Central ray of the primary beam*
*Direct the x-ray beam perpendicular to the cassette,
with the central ray centered at the level of T 10.*

■ *Notice*
*Stretch the thoracic limbs cranially and the
pelvic limbs caudally.*

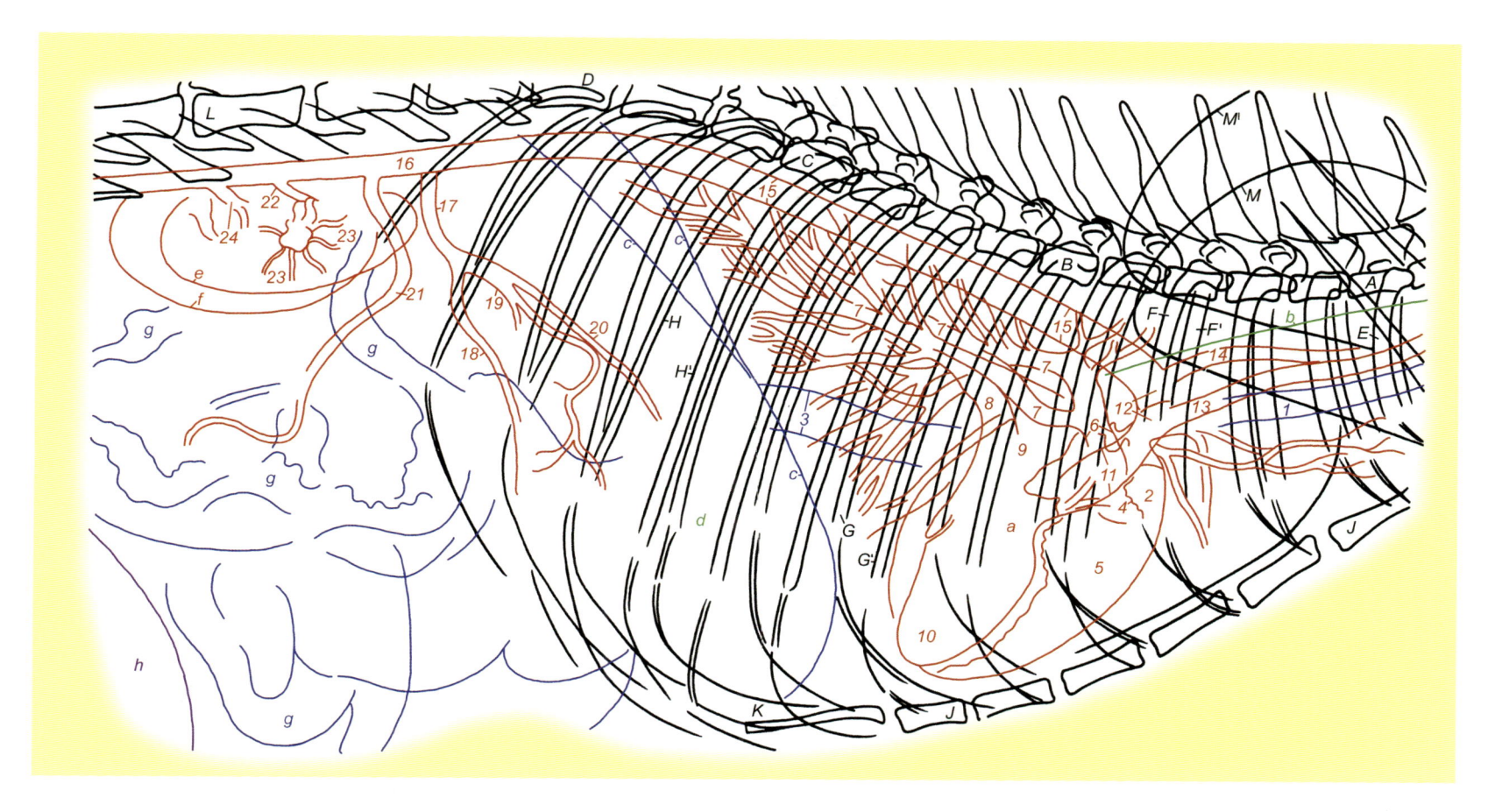

5.4 Angiokardiographie – Angiocardiography ■ latero-lateral

- **A** T I
- **B** T VI
- **C** T X
- **D** T XIII
- **E** Os costale I
- **F** Os costale IV, F´ plattenfern – *next to the tube*
- **G** Os costale VII, G´ plattenfern – *next to the tube*
- **H** Os costale X, H´ plattenfern – *next to the tube*
- **J** Sternebrae
- **K** Processus xiphoideus
- **L** L III
- **M** Scapula, M´ plattenfern – *next to the tube*

- **a** Cor
  - 1 Vena cava cranialis
  - 2 Auricula dextra
  - 3 Vena cava caudalis
  - 4 Ostium atrioventriculare dextrum
  - 5 Ventriculus dexter
  - 6 Truncus pulmonalis
  - 7 Aa. pulmonales
  - 8 Vv. pulmonales
  - 9 Atrium sinistrium
  - 10 Ventriculus sinister
  - 11 Bulbus aortae
  - 12 Arcus aortae
  - 13 Truncus brachiocephalicus
  - 14 A. subclavia sinistra
  - 15 Aorta thoracica
  - 16 Aorta abdominalis
  - 17 A. coeliaca
  - 18 A. lienalis
  - 19 A. gastrica sinistra
  - 20 A. hepatica
  - 21 A. mesenterica cranialis
  - 22 A. renalis dextra
  - 23 Aa. interlobares
  - 24 A. renalis sinistra

- **b** Trachea
- **c** Diaphragma
- **d** Hepar
- **e** Ren dexter
- **f** Ren sinister
- **g** Darmschlingen, zum Teil gashaltig – *intestinal loops, partly filled with gas*
- **h** gravider Uterus – *pregnant uterus*

6 Abdomen – Abdomen

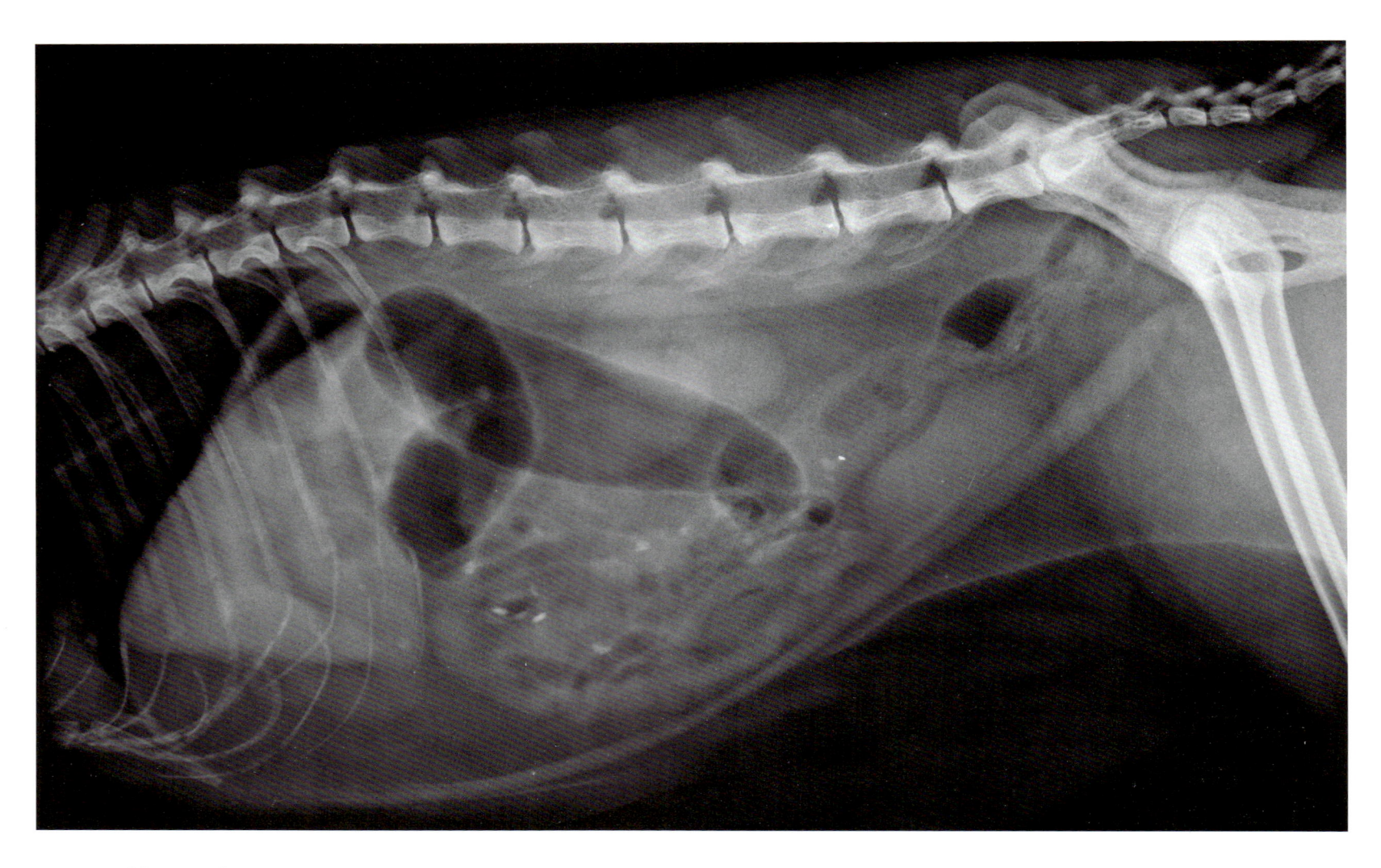

Abb. 6.1 Abdomen, liegend, latero-lateral,
Katze
(Verkleinerung von 24 × 30 cm)

Fig. 6.1 Abdomen, recumbent, latero-lateral,
Cat
(reduced from 24 × 30 cm)

■ **Ziel**
Übersichtsaufnahme der Bauchorgane, normalerweise in rechter Seitenlage; linke Seitenlage zur besonderen Beachtung des Canalis pyloricus, des Pylorus und des Duodenum ascendens.

■ **Zentralstrahl**
Auf die Regio abdominis lateralis, je nach Fragestellung:

Übersicht und **Darm:** ventral von L3
Magen: in der Mitte der 12. Rippe
Nieren: ventral von L3, am Übergang vom dorsalen zum mittleren Drittel der Bauchwand
Harnblase: ventral von L7
Lendenwirbelsäule: auf L3

■ **Beachte**
Die Medianebene soll parallel zur Kassette gelagert sein, bei fettleibigen Katzen kann dies durch Unterlegen eines Schaumgummikeils erreicht werden; die Beckengliedmaßen durch kaudales Strecken aus dem Aufnahmebereich ziehen.

■ *Objective*
To obtain a radiograph of the abdominal organs, normally performed in right lateral recumbency; left lateral recumbency is selected to image the canalis pyloricus, the pylorus and the ascending duodenum.

■ *Central ray of the primary beam*
Center the x-ray beam on the lateral abdominal region, depending on the clinical problem:

Survey *and* ***intestine:*** *ventral of L3*
Stomach: *in the middle of the 12th rib*
Kidneys: *ventral of L3, in the transition of the dorsal and middle thirds*
Urinary bladder: *ventral of L7*
Lumbar vertebral column: *on L3*

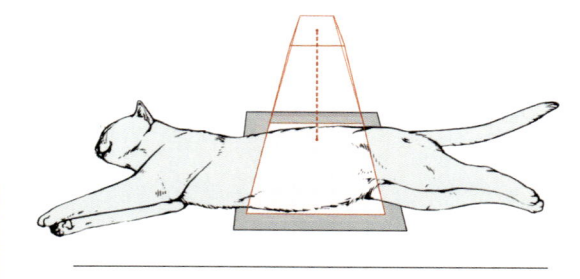

Abb. 6.1 Lagerung zur Aufnahme des Abdomens. Latero-lateral.

Fig. 6.1 Positioning of the abdomen. Latero-lateral.

■ *Notice*
Align the cassette parallel to the median plane, use a foam rubber wedge in obese patients, stretch the pelvic limbs caudally.

6.1 Abdomen – Abdomen ■ latero-lateral

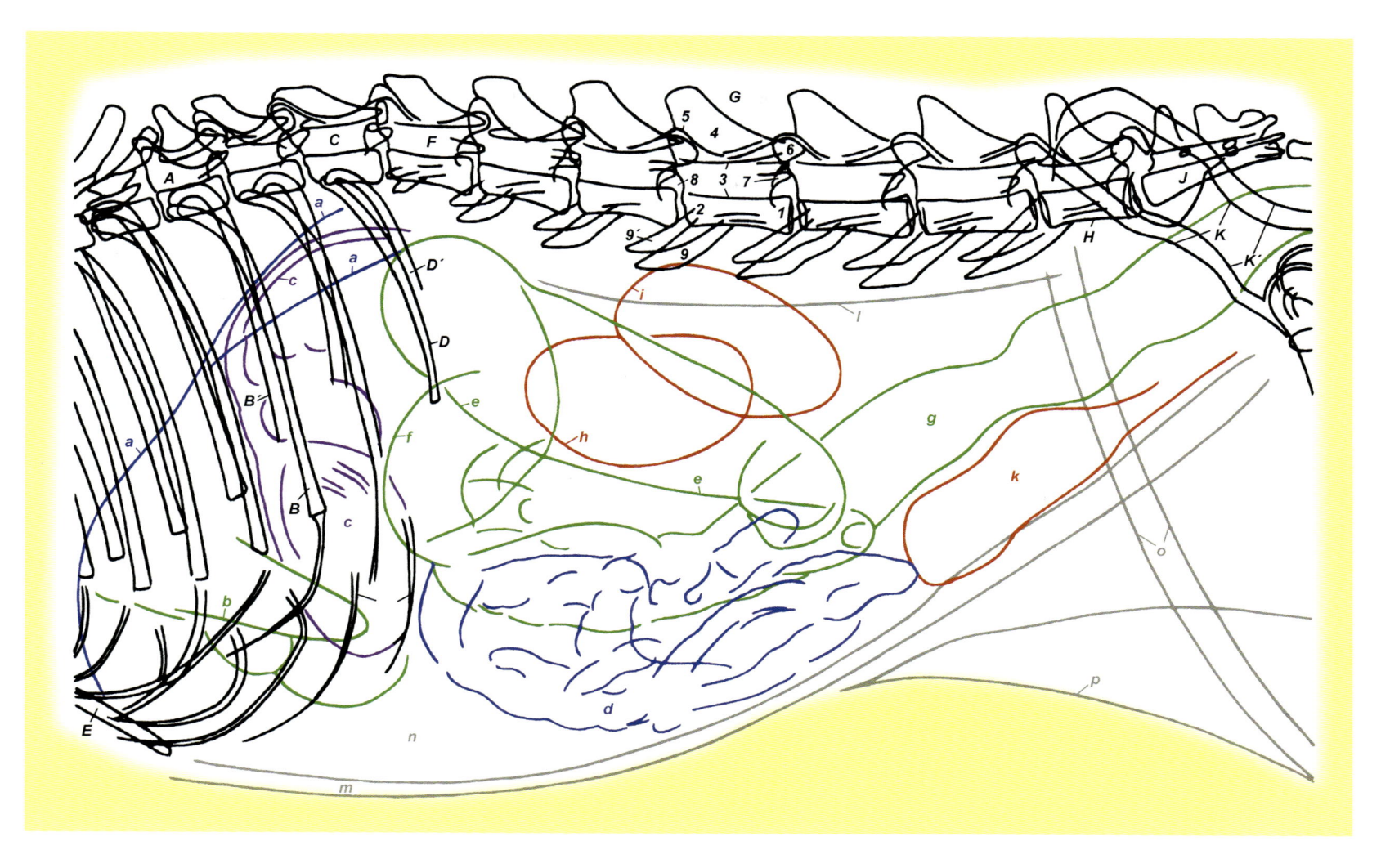

A T XI

B Os costale XI

C T XIII

D Os costale XIII, D´ plattenfern – *next to the tube*

E Processus xiphoideus

F L I

G L IV
   1 Facies terminalis cranialis
   2 Facies terminalis caudalis
   3 Foramen vertebrale
   4 Processus spinosus
   5 Processus mamilloarticularis
   6 Processus articularis caudalis
   7 Processus accessorius
   8 Foramen intervertebrale
   9 Processus transversus, 9´ plattenfern – *next to the tube*

H L VII

J Os sacrum

K Os ilium, K´ plattenfern – *next to the tube*

a **Diaphragma**

b **Hepar**

c **Ventriculus**

d **Jejunum**

e **Colon ascendens**

f **Colon transversum**

g **Colon descendens**

h **Ren dexter**

i **Ren sinister**

k **Vesica urinaria**

l innere Lendenmuskulatur, ventrale Begrenzung – *inner lumbar muscles, ventral border*

m ventrale Bauchwand – *ventral abdominal wall*

n Corpus adiposum

o Oberschenkelmuskulatur, kraniale Begrenzung – *cranial border of the femoral muscles*

p Plica lateris, Kniefalte – *fold of the flank*

6 Abdomen – Abdomen

Abb. 6.2 Abdomen, ventro-dorsal,
Katze
(Verkleinerung von 24 × 30 cm)

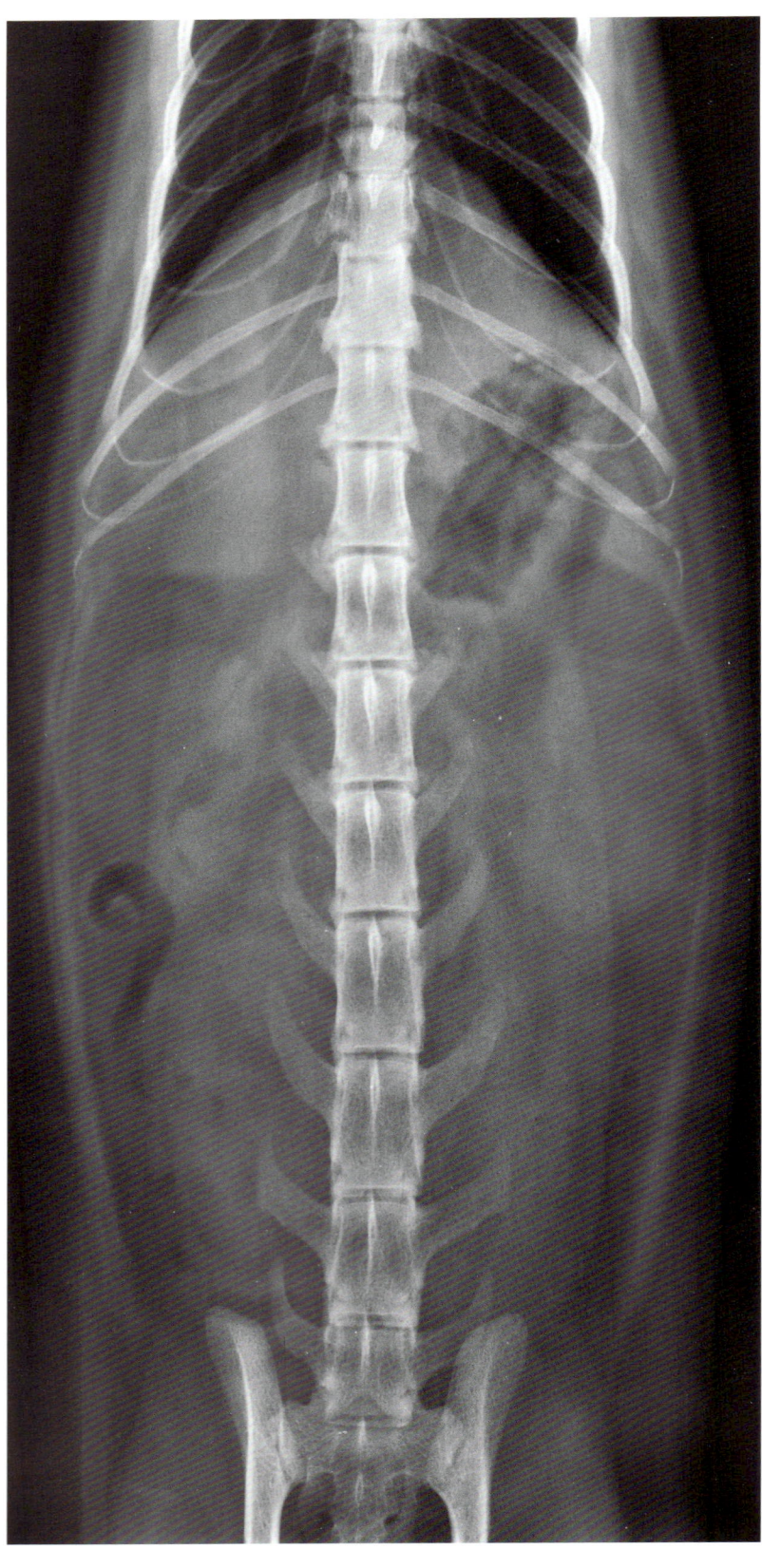

Fig. 6.2 Abdomen, ventro-dorsal,
Cat
(reduced from 24 × 30 cm)

■ **Ziel**
Darstellung der Bauchorgane.

■ **Zentralstrahl**
Senkrecht zur Kassette, auf die Medianebene, je nach Fragestellung:

Übersicht, Darm und **Nieren:** in Höhe des 2. Lendenwirbels
Magen: in Höhe des 12. Brustwirbels
Harnblase: in Höhe des 7. Lendenwirbels
Lendenwirbelsäule: in Höhe des 3. Lendenwirbels

■ **Objective**
To image the abdominal organs.

■ **Central ray of the primary beam**
Direct the x-ray beam perpendicular to the cassette, with the central ray centered on the median plane, depending on the clinical problem:

***Survey*, intestine** and **kidneys:** *at the level of L 2*
Stomach: *at the level of T 12*
Urinary bladder: *at the level of L 7*
Lumbar vertebral column: *at the level of L 3*

■ **Beachte**
Symmetrische Streckung der Schultergliedmaßen nach vorn und der Beckengliedmaßen nach hinten, keine Verkantung in der Längsachse.
Seitenbezeichnung nicht vergessen!

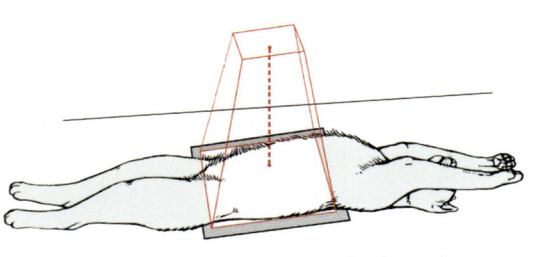

Abb. 6.2 Lagerung zur Aufnahme des Abdomens. Ventro-dorsal.

Fig. 6.2 Positioning of the abdomen. Ventro-dorsal.

■ **Notice**
Symmetric extension of the thoracic limbs cranially and the pelvic limbs caudally, do not tilt.
Do not forget the L/R mark!

6.2 Abdomen – Abdomen ■ ventro-dorsal

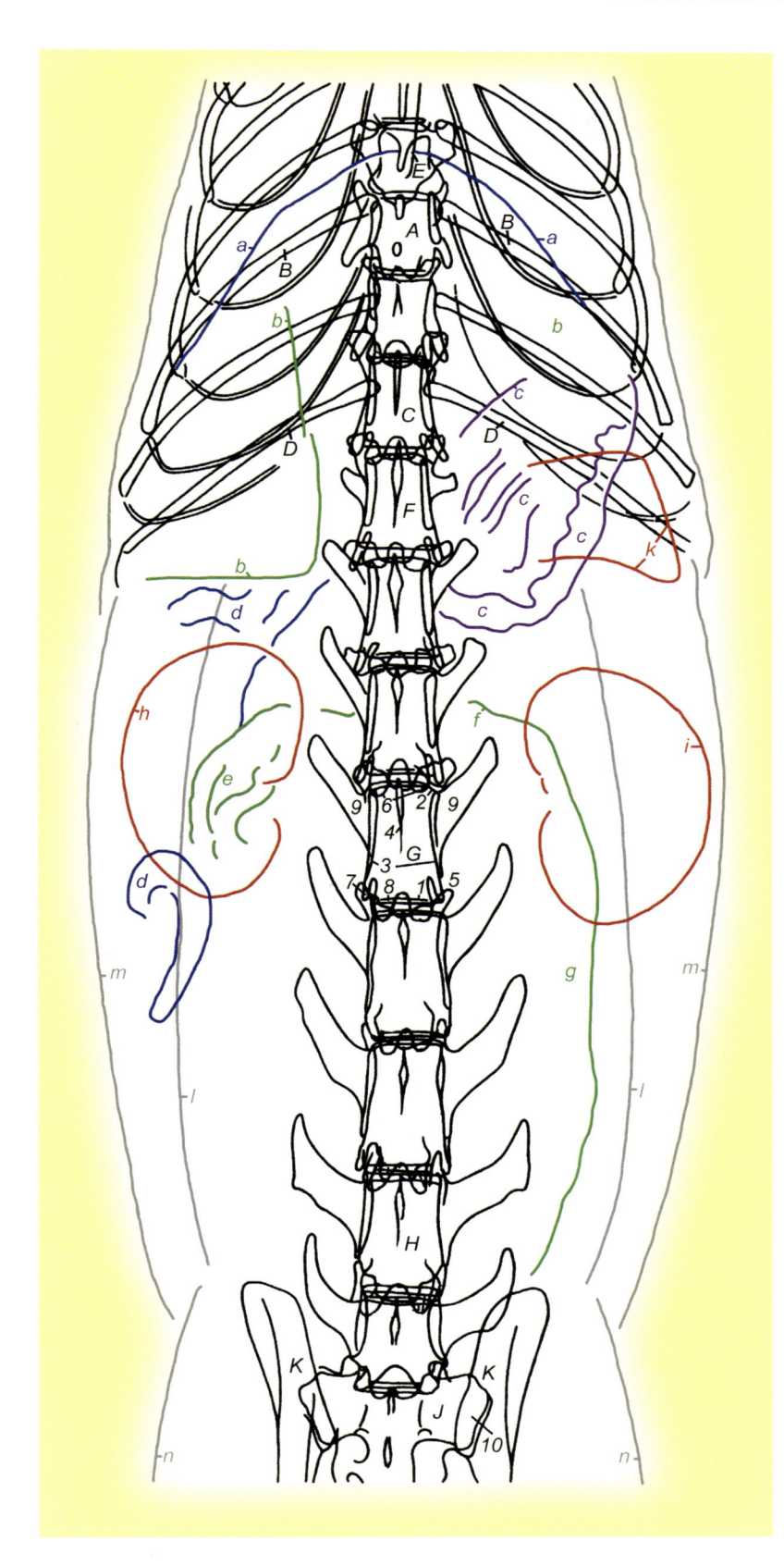

A   T XI

B   Os costale XI

C   T XIII

D   Os costale XIII

E   Processus xiphoideus

F   L I

G   L IV
    1   Facies terminalis caudalis
    2   Facies terminalis cranialis
    3   Foramen vertebrale
    4   Processus spinosus
    5   Processus articularis caudalis
    6   Processus articularis cranialis
    7   Processus accessorius
    8   Spatium interarcuale
    9   Processus transversus

H   L VII

J   Os sacrum
    10   Ala ossis sacri

K   Os ilium

a   **Diaphragma**

b   **Hepar**

c   **Ventriculus**

d   **Jejunum**

e   **Colon ascendens**

f   **Colon transversum**

g   **Colon descendens**

h   **Ren dexter**

i   **Ren sinister**

k   **Lien**

l   Stammmuskulatur, laterale Begrenzung – *muscles of the trunk, lateral border*

m   laterale Bauchwand – *lateral abdominal wall*

n   Gesäßmuskulatur, laterale Begrenzung – *lateral border of the gluteal muscles*

Beachte: Diese Katze hat 8 Lendenwirbel. –
Note: This cat has 8 lumbar vertebrae.

Ösophaguskontrolle, Magen-Darm-Kontrastuntersuchung

Vorbereitung

Abgesehen von einer dringlich notwendigen Untersuchung, wie bei Ileusverdacht, sollte eine Magen-Darm-Passage in nüchternem Zustand vorgenommen werden (12 Stunden fasten, eventuell ist eine Stunde vor der Untersuchung ein Reinigungseinlauf durchzuführen). Als Sedativum kann Acepromacin 30 Minuten vor der Kontrastmitteluntersuchung eingesetzt werden.

Kontrastmittel

Für die Katze ist Prontobario® (Bariumsulfat mit peristaltikförderndem Zusatz) ein sehr vorteilhaftes Kontrastmittel, es wird relativ gern aufgenommen, seine Entleerung aus dem Magen in den Darm erfolgt meist ohne Verzögerung. Bei Bariumsulfat-Suspension allein kann die Magenentleerung wegen Aufregung über Stunden sistieren; bei Exsikkose kann Bariumsulfat im Darm eingedickt werden und verklumpen.

Nicht empfehlenswert ist das jodhaltige Kontrastmittel Gastrografin, es hat eine geringe Dichte und einen schlechten Geschmack; als hyperosmolares Kontrastmittel nimmt es über den Darm Körperflüssigkeiten auf, wodurch sich die Dichte weiter vermindert und eine etwaige Exsikkose weiter verstärkt wird.

Die Eingabe erfolgt seitlich über die Mundspalte mit einer Spritze mit Metallkonus, um ein Durchbeißen zu verhindern, oder mittels Magensonde; hiermit kann auch Luft insuffliert werden.

Kontrastmittelmenge: 10–30 ml Suspension Prontobario®, falls unbedingt notwendig kann ein jodhaltiges Kontrastmittel in einer Dosierung von 2 ml/kg Körpergewicht gegeben werden.

Untersuchungstechnik

Ösophaguskontrolle: latero-laterale Hals- bzw. Thoraxaufnahme im Anschluss an die Per-os-Kontrastmitteleingabe. Merke: Die Speiseröhre verfügt kaudal des Herzens über Längs- und Ringmuskulatur, wodurch sich das typische „Fischgrätenmuster" ergibt.

Magen: Grundbilderpaar (latero-lateral, ventro-dorsal), bei spezieller Fragestellung den Magen betreffend besser 4 Aufnahmeebenen sofort nach Kontrastmitteleingabe; die Entleerung des Magens erfolgt 5 Minuten nach der Eingabe und ist nach 2 Stunden beendet.

Darmpassage: Kontrollen nach 10, 20, 30 und 60 Minuten, eventuell weiterhin in stündlichen Abständen, bis der Dünndarm passiert und das Caecum erreicht ist; Aufnahmen latero-lateral und ventro-dorsal. Das Caecum erscheint fingerförmig. Kontrast kann hier längere Zeit liegen bleiben; dieses Bild darf nicht mit einer Aufstauung im Dünndarm verwechselt werden.

Das Duodenum ist bei gesunden Katzen nach 5 Minuten zur Gänze dargestellt, nach nach 2–2,5 Stunden das Caecum, nach 4 Stunden das Colon descendens. Jodhaltige Kontrastmittel in wässriger Lösung erreichen das Caecum nach 30–45 Minuten.

Irrigoskopie: Nach Entleerung des Enddarms können bei der sedierten Katze 30–50 ml einer dickflüssigen, körperwarmen Bariumsulfat-Suspension mittels Ballonkatheters appliziert werden. Grundbilderpaar (latero-lateral, ventro-dorsal) anfertigen.

Esophageal, gastric and intestinal contrast study

Preparation

Except in emergency situations (e.g., ileus), a gastric and intestinal contrast study is be performed in patients that have had food withheld for 12 hours. Eventually a cleansing enema, one hour before the contrast examination, is performed. For sedation, acepromacine can be administered 30 minutes before the contrast administration.

Contrast media

In cats, Prontobario® (barium sulfate suspension with a peristalsis stimulating additive) is the preferred contrast medium. It is well accepted by the patient and is promptly emptied from the stomach into the duodenum. In contrast, the patient's excitement can cause barium suspensions to be held in the stomach for hours. Additionally, barium suspensions can be dried and congealed in dehydrated patients. Gastrografin is not recommended because of its low density, bad taste, and hyperosmolarity. Gastrografin absorbs fluid from the gut, leading to further decreasing density of the contrast medium and increasing dehydration of the patient.

The positive contrast medium is administered into the cheek-pouch using a syringe with a metallic cone in order to prevent break-down of the syringe. Room air can be administered using a gastric tube. Contrast dosage is 10–30 ml of Prontobario® or – if needed – an iodinated contrast medium in a dose of 2 ml/kg of body weight.

Technique

Esophageal control: laterolateral view of the neck and thorax immediately following the oral contrast administration. Be aware that, due to the transition to smooth muscle in the feline esophagus caudal to the heart, this portion of the esophagram is normally imaged as a "herring-bone" mucosal pattern.

Stomach: routinely two radiographs at a 90-degree angle (ventrodorsal, and left-right lateral) are performed. A complete examination of the stomach includes 4 projections following the contrast administration. Gastric emptying typically begins 5 minutes after the oral contrast administration, and complete emptying usually requires about 2 hours.

Intestinal passage: In a routine upper GI study, radiographs are made at 10, 20, 30 and 60 minutes following contrast administration, and, if needed, every other hour, until the contrast has reached the cecum. Laterolateral and ventrodorsal projections are performed. The normal feline cecum has a diameter of a finger and should be differentiated from an ileal obstruction.

In normal cats, the duodenum can be imaged 5 minutes after oral contrast administration, the cecum at 2 to 2.5 hours, and the ascending colon at about 4 hours. Iodinated contrast medium reaches the cecum about 30 to 45 minutes after oral contrast administration.

Irrigoscopy (Barium Enema): After a cleansing enema, 30 to 50 ml of a viscous barium sulfate suspension, warmed to body temperature, is infused into the rectum using a balloon catheter. Laterolateral and ventrodorsal projections are performed.

6 Abdomen – Abdomen

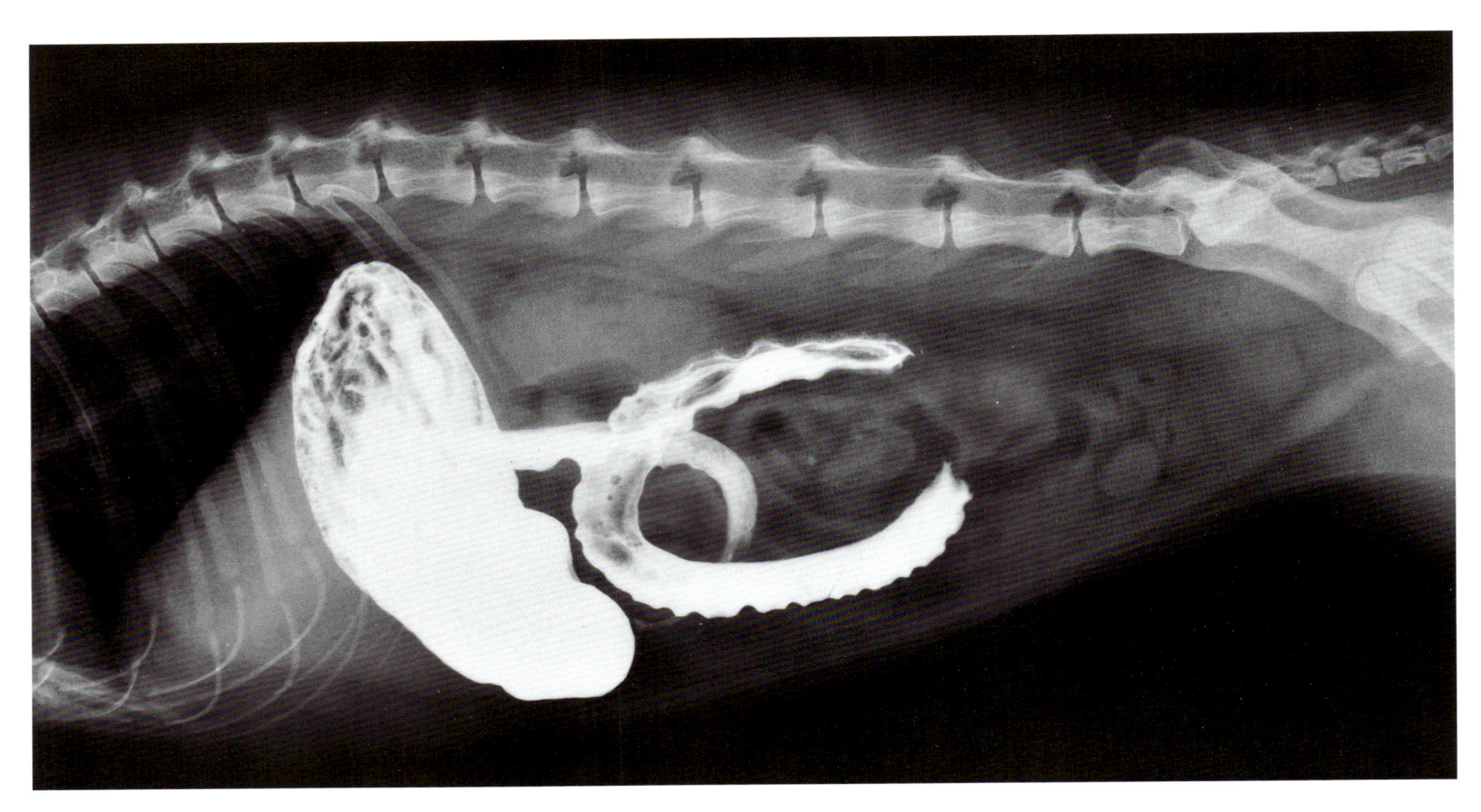

Abb. 6.3 Magen-Darm-Kontrast, liegend, latero-lateral
(Barium sulfuricum),
Katze
(Verkleinerung von 15 × 40 cm)

Fig. 6.3 Stomach-intestine-contrast, recumbent, latero-lateral
(Barium sulphate),
Cat
(reduced from 15 × 40 cm)

■ **Ziel**
Kontrastdarstellung des Magens und proximaler Abschnitte des Dünndarms.

■ **Zentralstrahl**
Senkrecht zur Kassette, auf die Regio abdominis lateralis in Höhe des 3. Lendenwirbels.

■ **Beachte**
Die Medianebene soll parallel zur Kassette gelagert sein, bei fettleibigen Katzen kann dies durch Unterlegen eines Schaumgummikeils erreicht werden; die Beckengliedmaßen nach kaudal strecken.

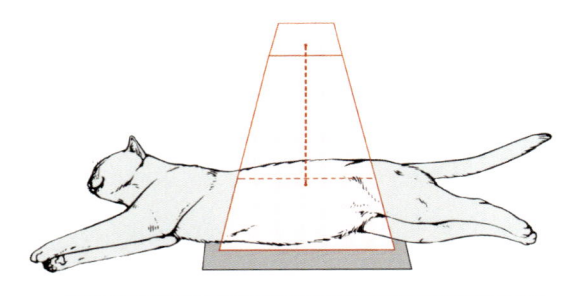

Abb. 6.3 Lagerung zur Aufnahme des Abdomens. Liegend. Latero-lateral.

Fig. 6.3 Positioning of the abdomen. Recumbent. Latero-lateral.

■ *Objective*
To obtain a contrast radiographic study of the stomach and proximal part of the small intestine.

■ *Central ray of the primary beam*
Direct the central ray of the x-ray beam perpendicular to the cassette, centered on the lateral abdominal region, at the level of L 3.

■ *Notice*
Align the cassette parallel to the median plane, use a foam rubber wedge in adipose patients, stretch pelvic limbs caudally.

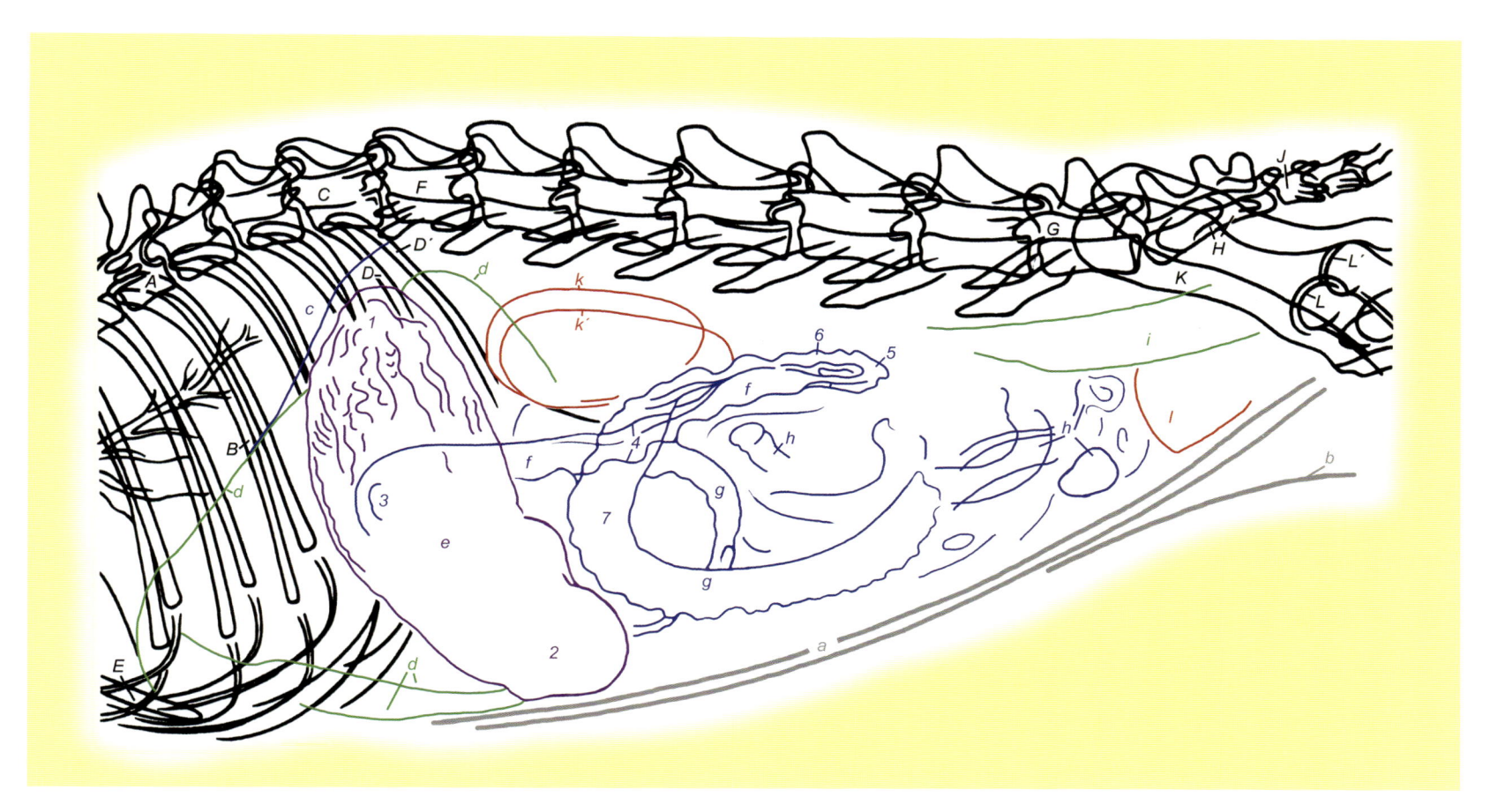

6.3 Kontrast, Magen, Dünndarm – contrast, stomach, intestine ■ latero-lateral

- A T X
- B Os costale X
- C T XIII
- D Os costale XIII, D´ plattenfern – next to the tube
- E Processus xiphoideus
- F L I
- G L VII
- H Os sacrum
- J Co I
- K Os ilium

- L Caput ossis femoris, L´ plattenfern – next to the tube

- a ventrale Bauchwand – ventral abdominal wall
- b Plica lateris, Kniefalte – fold of the flank
- c Diaphragma
- d Hepar
- e Ventriculus
  - 1 Fundus ventriculi
  - 2 Corpus ventriculi
- f Duodenum
  - 3 Pars cranialis
  - 4 Pars descendens
  - 5 Pars transversa
  - 6 Pars ascendens
  - 7 Flexura duodenojejunalis
- g Jejunum (zum Teil mit Kontrastmittel – partly with contrast medium)
- h Jejunum (zum Teil gashaltig – partly filled with gas)
- i Colon descendens
- k Ren dexter
- k´ Ren sinister
- l Vesica urinaria

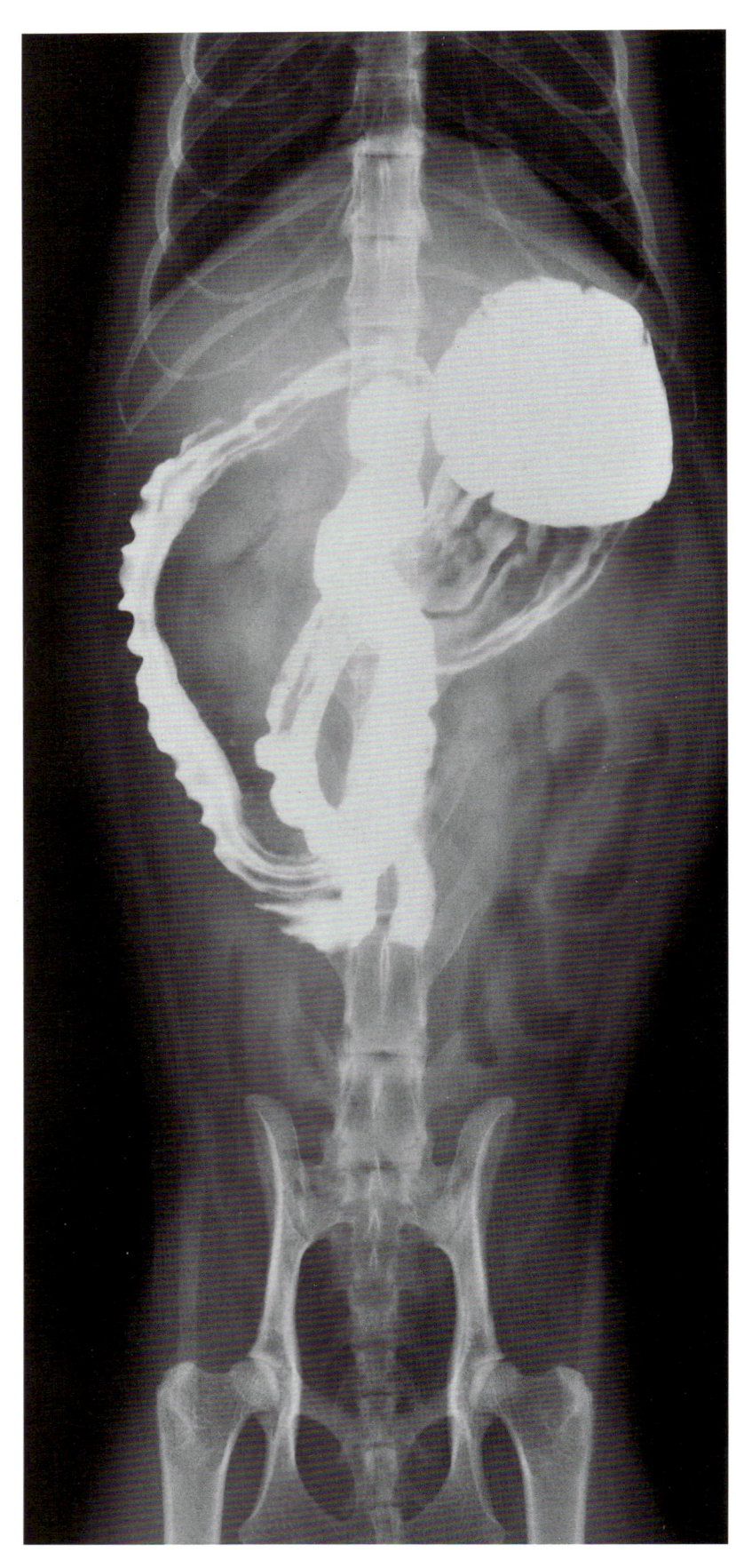

6 Abdomen – Abdomen

Abb. 6.4 Magen-Darm-Kontrast, ventro-dorsal
(Barium sulfuricum),
Katze
(Verkleinerung von 15 × 40 cm)

Fig. 6.4 Stomach-intestine-contrast, ventro-dorsal
(Barium sulphate),
Cat
(reduced from 15 × 40 cm)

■ **Ziel**
Übersichtsaufnahme der Bauchorgane, mit Kontrastdarstellung des Magens und des Dünndarms.

■ **Zentralstrahl**
Senkrecht zur Kassette, auf die Medianebene, in Höhe des 3. Lendenwirbels.

■ *Objective*
To obtain a ventro-dorsal contrast radiographic study of the stomach and small intestine.

■ *Central ray of the primary beam*
Direct the x-ray beam perpendicular to the cassette, with the central ray centered on the median plane, at the level of L 3.

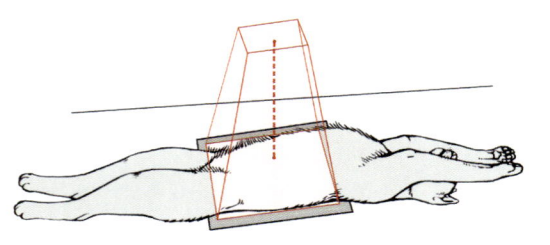

Abb. 6.4 Lagerung zur Aufnahme des Abdomens. Ventro-dorsal.

Fig. 6.4 Positioning of the abdomen. Ventro-dorsal.

■ **Beachte**
Lagerung kann durch Schaumgummikeile erreicht werden. Beckengliedmaße nach kaudal strecken.
Seitenbestimmung nicht vergessen!

■ *Notice*
*Positioning can be supported by foam rubber wedges, stretch pelvic limbs caudally.
Do not forget the L/R mark!*

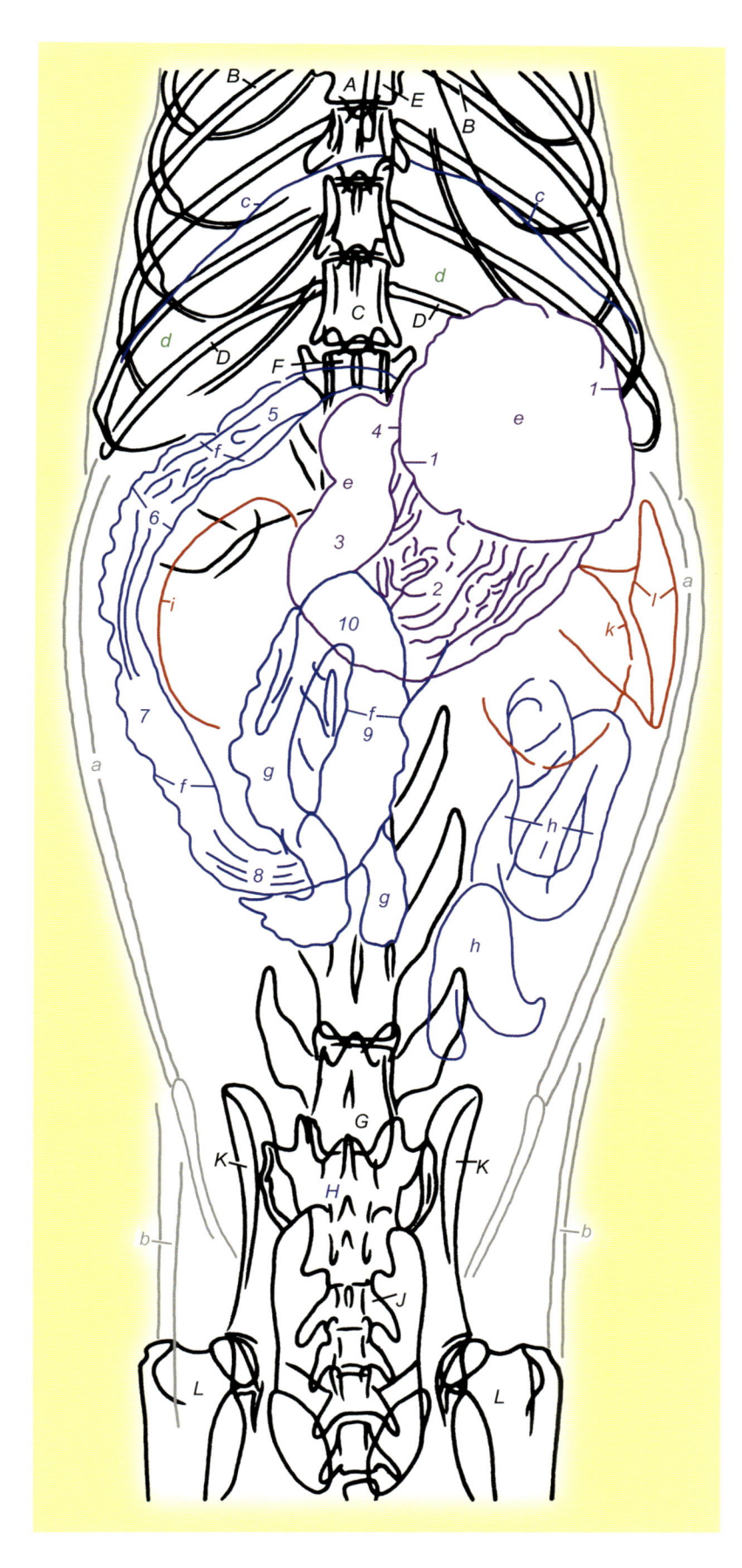

6.4 Kontrast, Magen, Dünndarm – contrast, stomach, intestine ■ ventro-dorsal

A T X

B Os costale X

C T XIII

D Os costale XIII

E Processus xiphoideus

F L I

G L VII

H Os sacrum

J Co I

K Os ilium

L Os femoris

a seitliche Bauchwand – *lateral abdominal wall*

b Plica lateris, Kniefalte – *fold of the flank*

c Diaphragma

d Hepar

e Ventriculus
  1 Fundus ventriculi
  2 Corpus ventriculi
  3 Pars pylorica
  4 Pylorus

f Duodenum (mit Kontrastmittel – *with contrast medium*)
  5 Pars cranialis
  6 Flexura duodeni cranialis
  7 Pars descendens
  8 Pars transversa
  9 Pars ascendens
  10 Flexura duodenojejunalis

g Jejunum (zum Teil mit Kontrastmittel – *partly filled with contrast medium*)

h Jejunum (zum Teil gashaltig – *partly filled with gas*)

i Ren dexter

k Ren sinister

l Lien

6 Abdomen – Abdomen

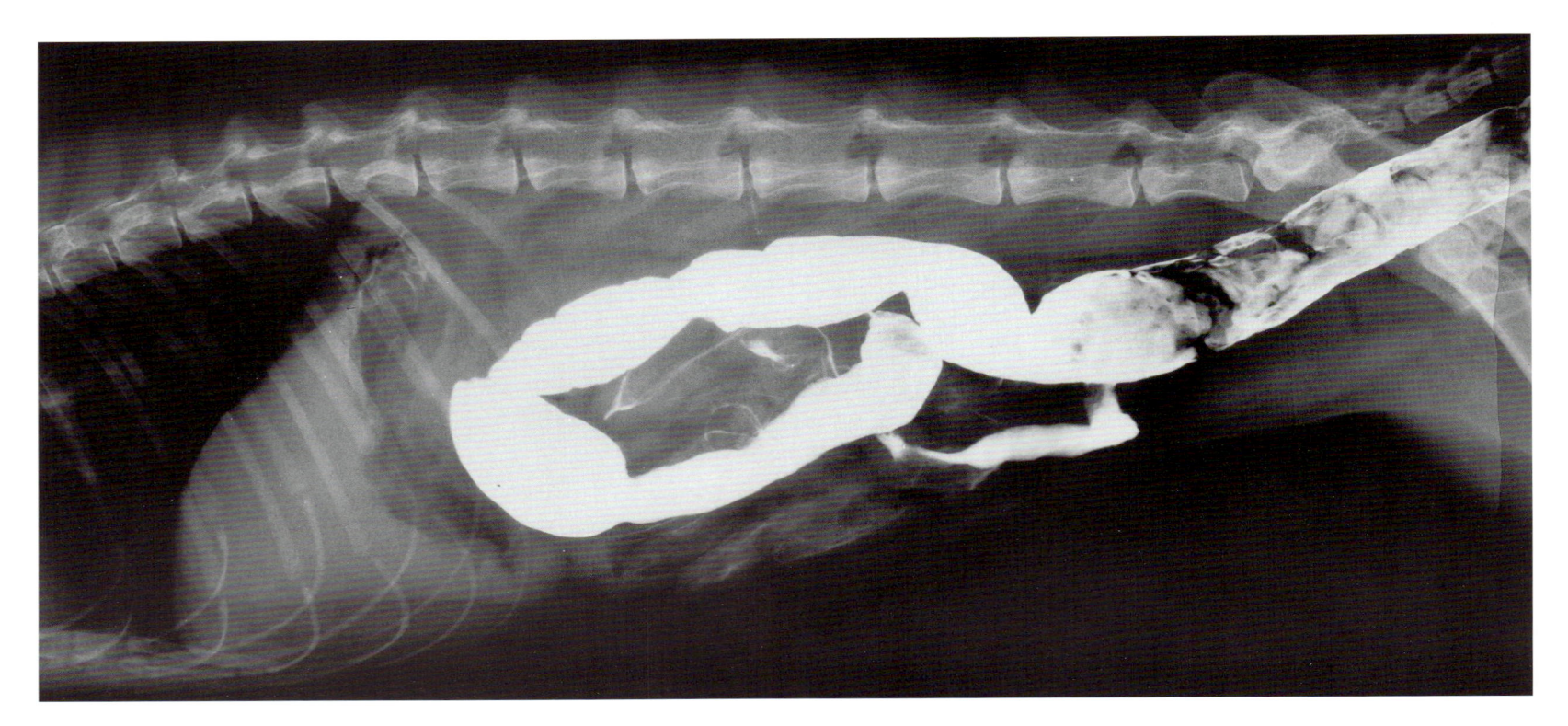

Abb. 6.5 Darm-Kontrast, liegend, latero-lateral
(Barium sulfuricum),
Katze
(Verkleinerung von 15 × 40 cm)

Fig. 6.5 Intestine-contrast, recumbent, latero-lateral
(Barium sulphate),
Cat
(reduced from 15 × 40 cm)

■ **Ziel**
Übersichtsaufnahme der Bauchorgane mit Kontrastdarstellung des Dickdarms.

■ **Zentralstrahl**
Senkrecht zur Kassette, auf die Regio abdominis lateralis in Höhe des 3. Lendenwirbels.

■ **Beachte**
Die Medianebene soll parallel zur Kassette gelagert sein, bei fettleibigen Katzen kann dies durch Unterlegen eines Schaumgummikeils erreicht werden; die Beckengliedmaßen nach kaudal strecken.

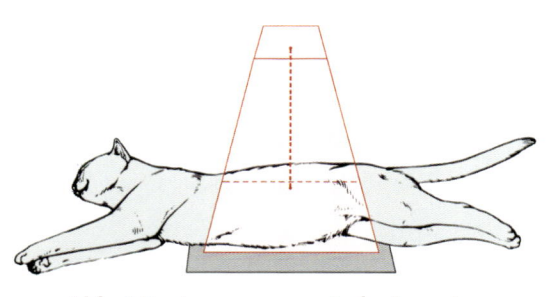

Abb. 6.5 Lagerung zur Aufnahme des Abdomens. Liegend. Latero-lateral.

Fig. 6.5 Positioning of the abdomen. Recumbent. Latero-lateral.

■ *Objective*
To obtain a lateral contrast radiographic study of the large intestine.

■ *Central ray of the primary beam*
Direct the x-ray beam perpendicular to the cassette, with the central ray centered on the lateral abdominal region, at the level of L3.

■ *Notice*
Align the cassette parallel to the median plane, use a foam rubber wedge in adipose patients, stretch pelvic limbs caudally.

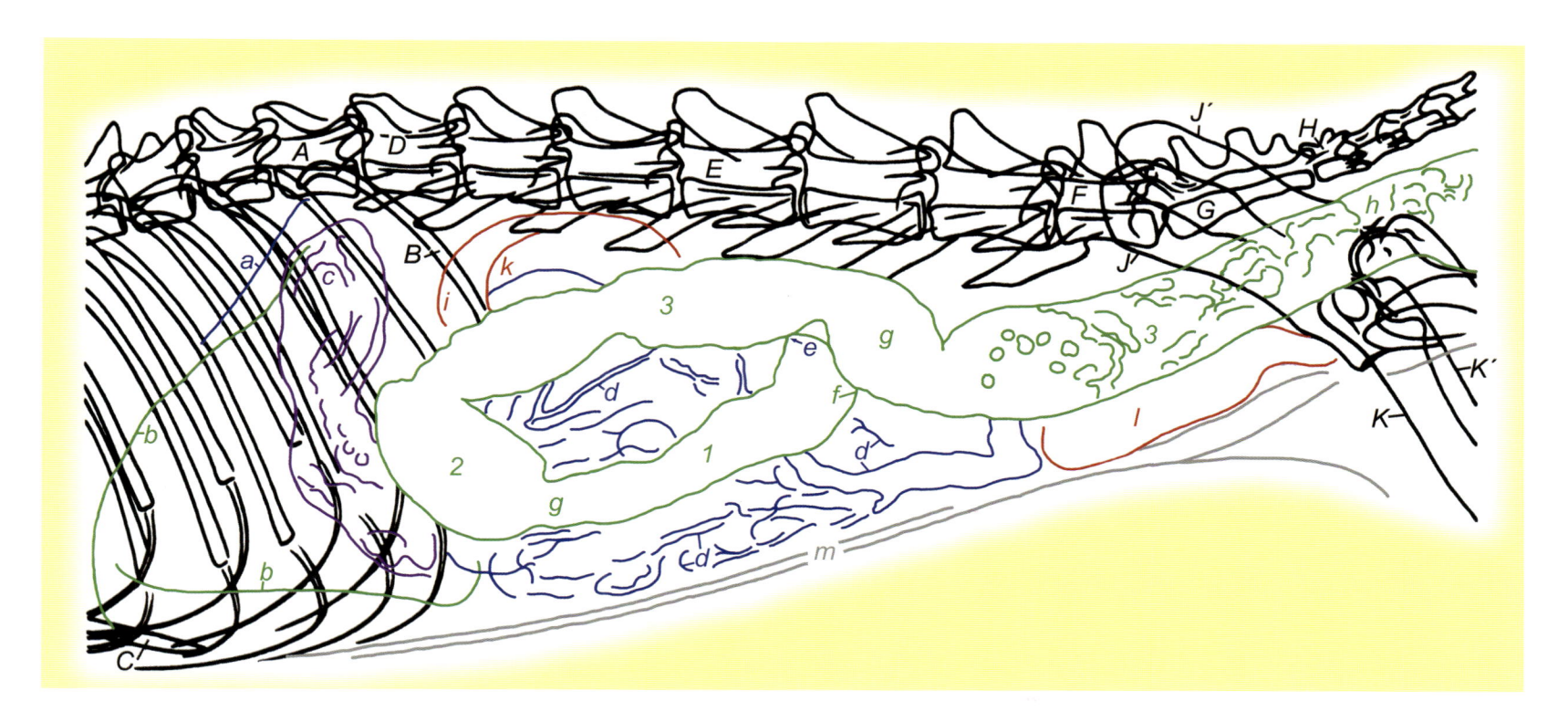

6.5 Kontrast, Darm – contrast, intestine ■ latero-lateral

- A T XIII
- B Os costale XIII
- C Processus xiphoideus
- D L I
- E L IV
- F L VII
- G Os sacrum
- H Co I
- J Os ilium, J´ plattenfern – *next to the tube*
- K Os femoris, K´ plattenfern – *next to the tube*

- a Diaphragma
- b Hepar
- c Fundus ventriculi mit Kontrastmittelresten – *with residual contrast medium*
- d Jejunumschlingen mit Kontrastmittelresten – *jejunal loops, with residual contrast medium*
- e Ileum
- f Caecum

- g **Colon**
    - 1 Colon ascendens
    - 2 Colon transversum
    - 3 Colon descendens
- h **Rectum**
- i **Ren dexter**
- k **Ren sinister**
- l **Vesica urinaria**
- m ventrale Bauchwand – *ventral abdominal wall*

6 Abdomen – Abdomen

**Abb. 6.6 Darm-Kontrast,
ventro-dorsal**
(Barium sulfuricum),
Katze
(Verkleinerung von 15 × 40 cm)

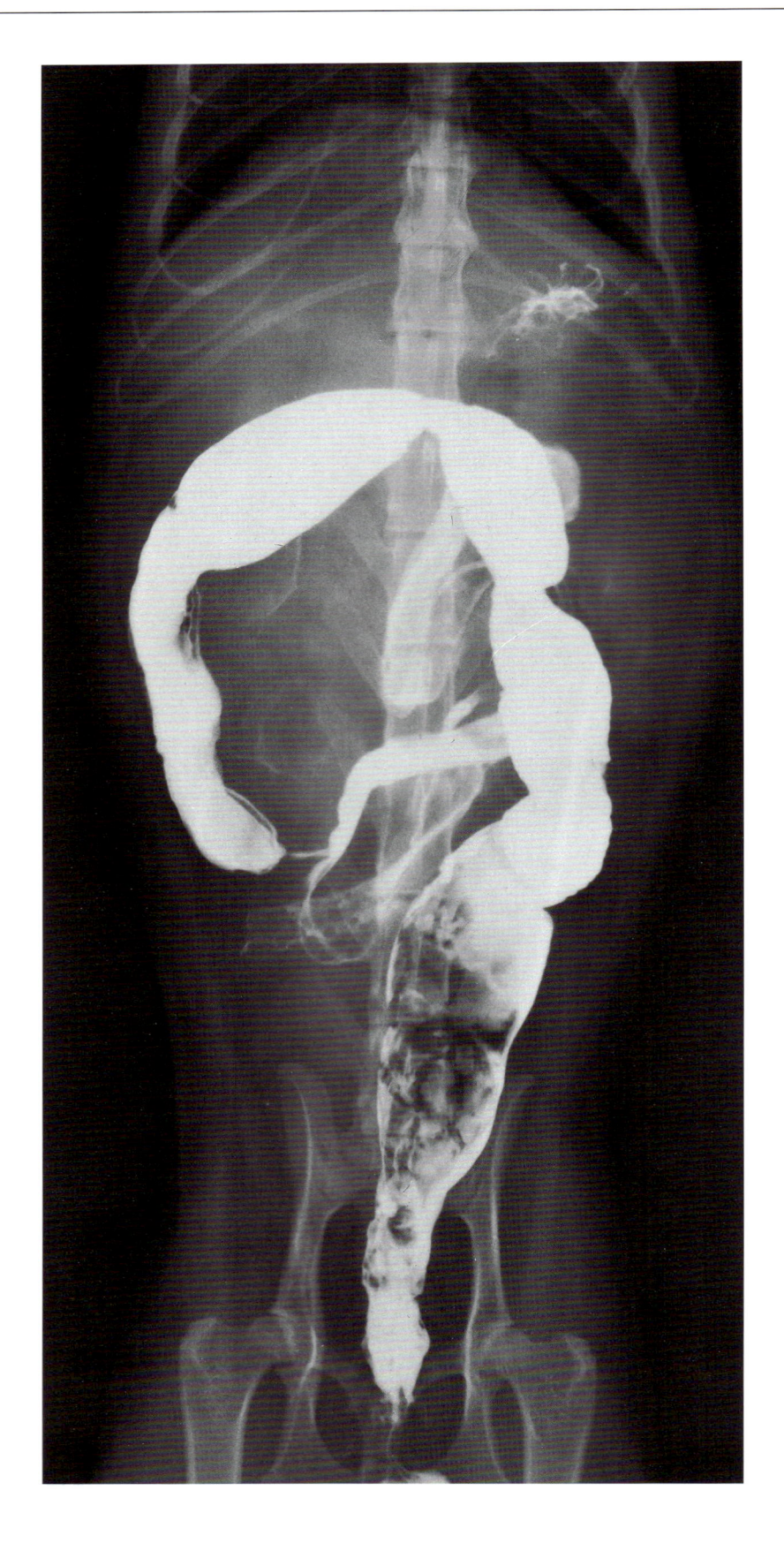

*Fig. 6.6 Intestine-contrast,
ventro-dorsal*
(Barium sulphate),
Cat
(reduced from 15 × 40 cm)

■ **Ziel**
Übersichtsaufnahme der Bauchorgane, mit Kontrastdarstellung des Dickdarms.

■ **Zentralstrahl**
Senkrecht zur Kassette, auf die Medianebene, in Höhe des 3. Lendenwirbels.

■ **Beachte**
Lagerung kann durch Schaumgummikeile erreicht werden. Beckengliedmaße nach kaudal strecken.
Seitenbestimmung nicht vergessen!

Abb. 6.6 Lagerung zur Aufnahme des Abdomens. Ventro-dorsal.

*Fig. 6.6 Positioning of the abdomen.
Ventro-dorsal.*

■ *Objective*
To obtain a ventro-dorsal contrast radiographic study of the large intestine.

■ *Central ray of the primary beam*
Direct the x-ray beam perpendicular to the cassette, with the central ray centered on the median plane, at the level of L 3.

■ *Notice*
*Positioning can be supported by foam rubber wedges, stretch pelvic limbs caudally.
Do not forget the L/R mark!*

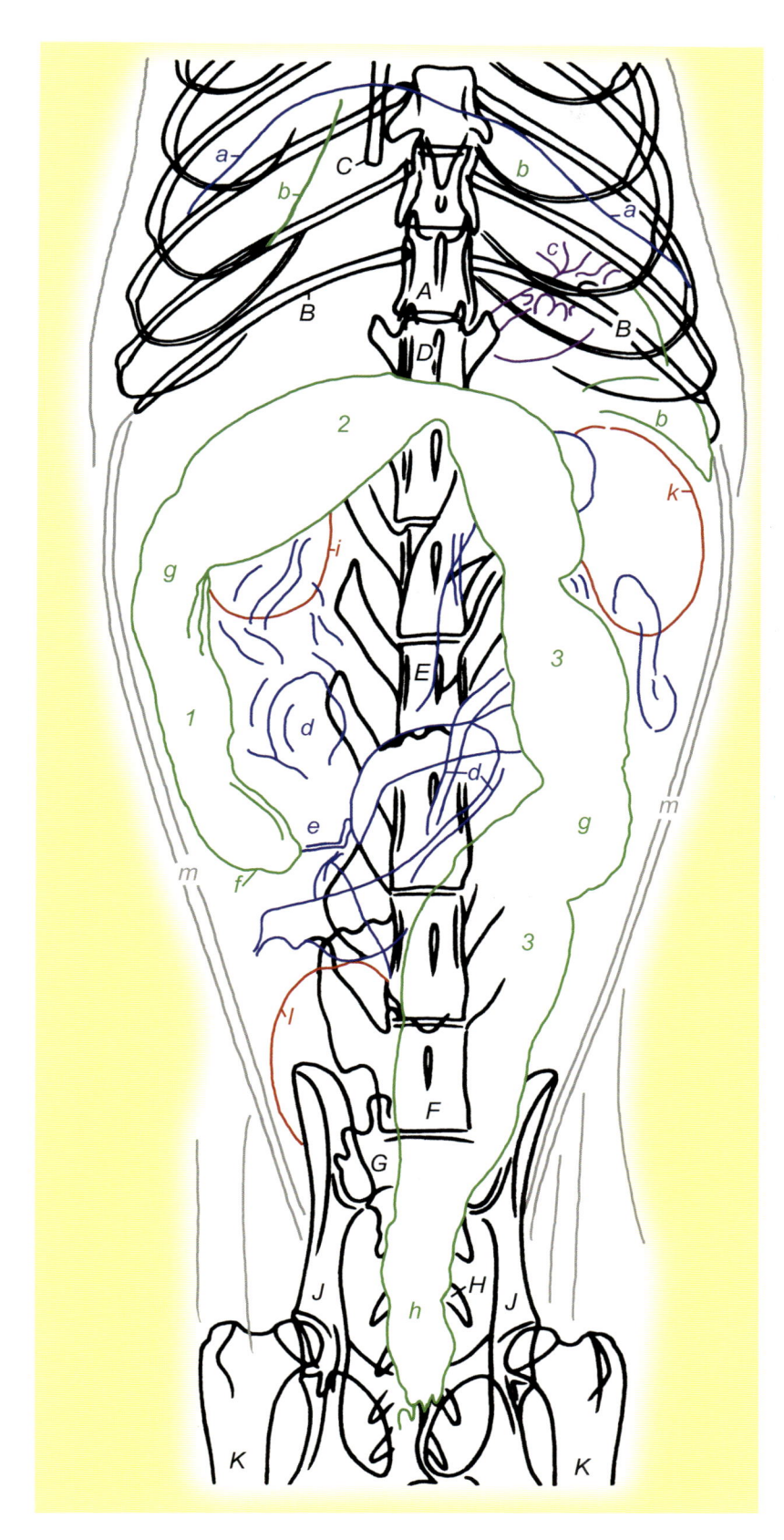

6.6 Kontrast, Dickdarm – contrast, intestine ■ ventro-dorsal

A   T XIII

B   Os costale XIII

C   Processus xiphoideus

D   L I

E   L IV

F   L VII

G   Os sacrum

H   Co I

J   Os ilium

K   Os femoris

a   Diaphragma

b   Hepar

c   **Fundus ventriculi mit Kontrastmittelresten** – *with residual contrast medium*

d   **Jejunumschlingen mit Kontrastmittelresten** – *jejunal loops with residual contrast medium*

e   Ileum

f   Caecum

g   Colon
    1   Colon ascendens
    2   Colon transversum
    3   Colon descendens

h   Rectum

i   Ren dexter

k   Ren sinister

l   Vesica urinaria

m   seitliche Bauchwand – *lateral abdominal wall*

103

6 Abdomen – Abdomen

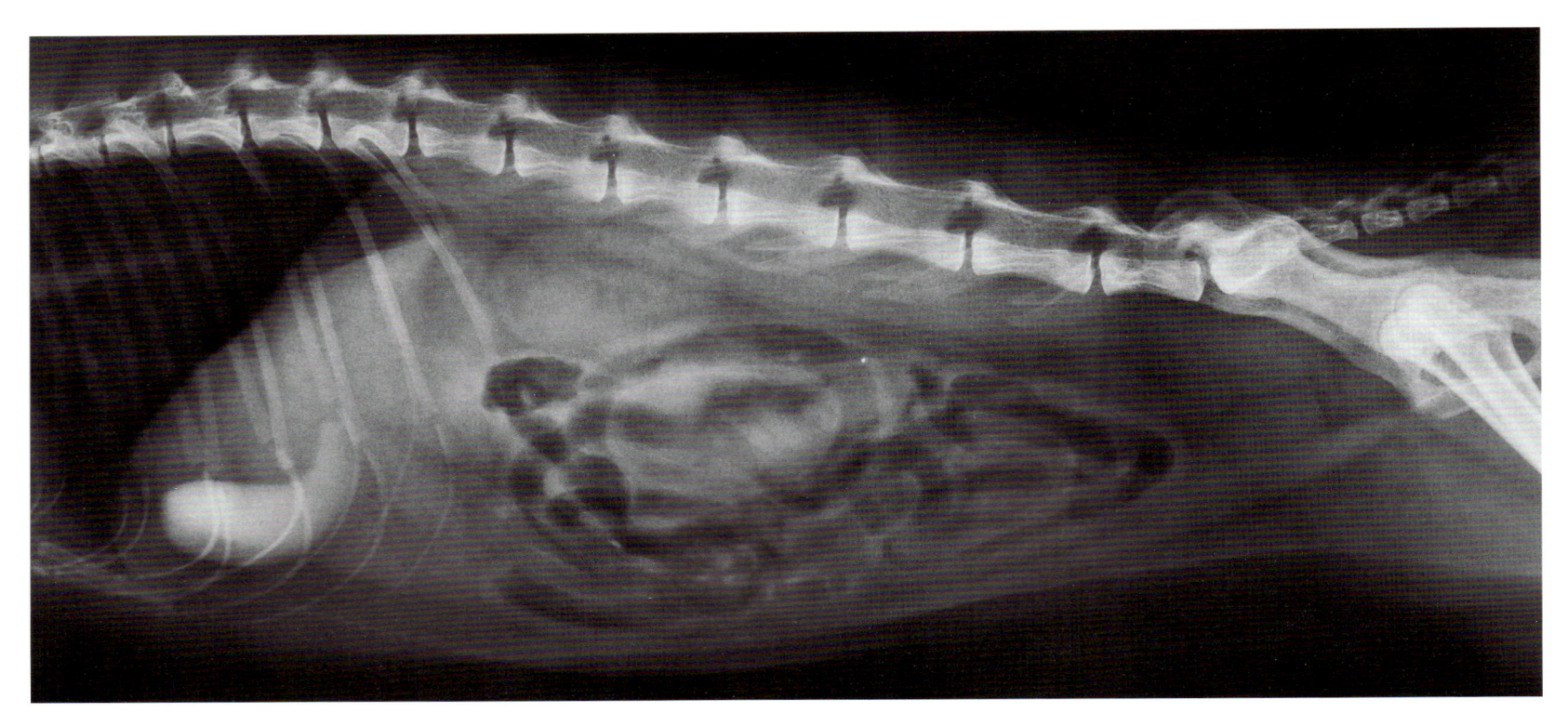

**Abb. 6.7 Gallenblasen-Darstellung,
liegend, latero-lateral**
(Biloptin®, Schering),
Katze
(Verkleinerung von 15 × 40 cm)

*Fig. 6.7 Gallbladder-contrast,
recumbent, latero-lateral*
(Biloptin®, Schering),
Cat
(reduced from 15 × 40 cm)

■ **Ziel**
Übersichtsaufnahme der Bauchorgane mit Kontrastdarstellung der Gallenblase.

■ **Zentralstrahl**
Senkrecht zur Kassette, auf die Regio abdominis lateralis, in Höhe des 3. Lendenwirbels.

■ **Beachte**
Lagerung kann durch Schaumgummikeile erreicht werden. Beckengliedmaße nach kaudal strecken.
Seitenbestimmung nicht vergessen!

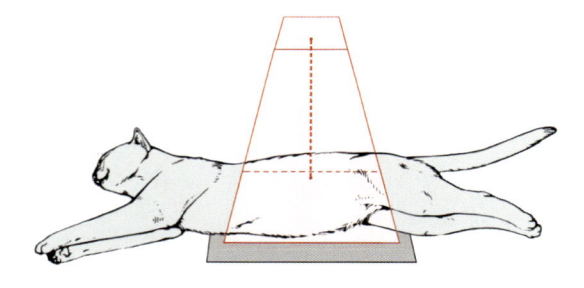

**Abb. 6.7 Lagerung zur Aufnahme des
Abdomens. Latero-lateral.**

**Diese Untersuchungstechnik wurde nahezu
vollständig durch die Sonographie ersetzt.**

*Fig. 6.7 Positioning of the abdomen.
Latero-lateral.*

*This technique was replaced nearly
completely by sonography.*

■ *Objective*
To obtain a lateral contrast radiographic study of the gallbladder.

■ *Central ray of the primary beam*
Direct the x-ray beam perpendicular to the cassette, with the central ray centered on the lateral abdominal region, at the level of L3.

■ *Notice*
*Positioning can be supported by foam rubber wedges, stretch pelvic limbs caudally.
Do not forget the L/R mark!*

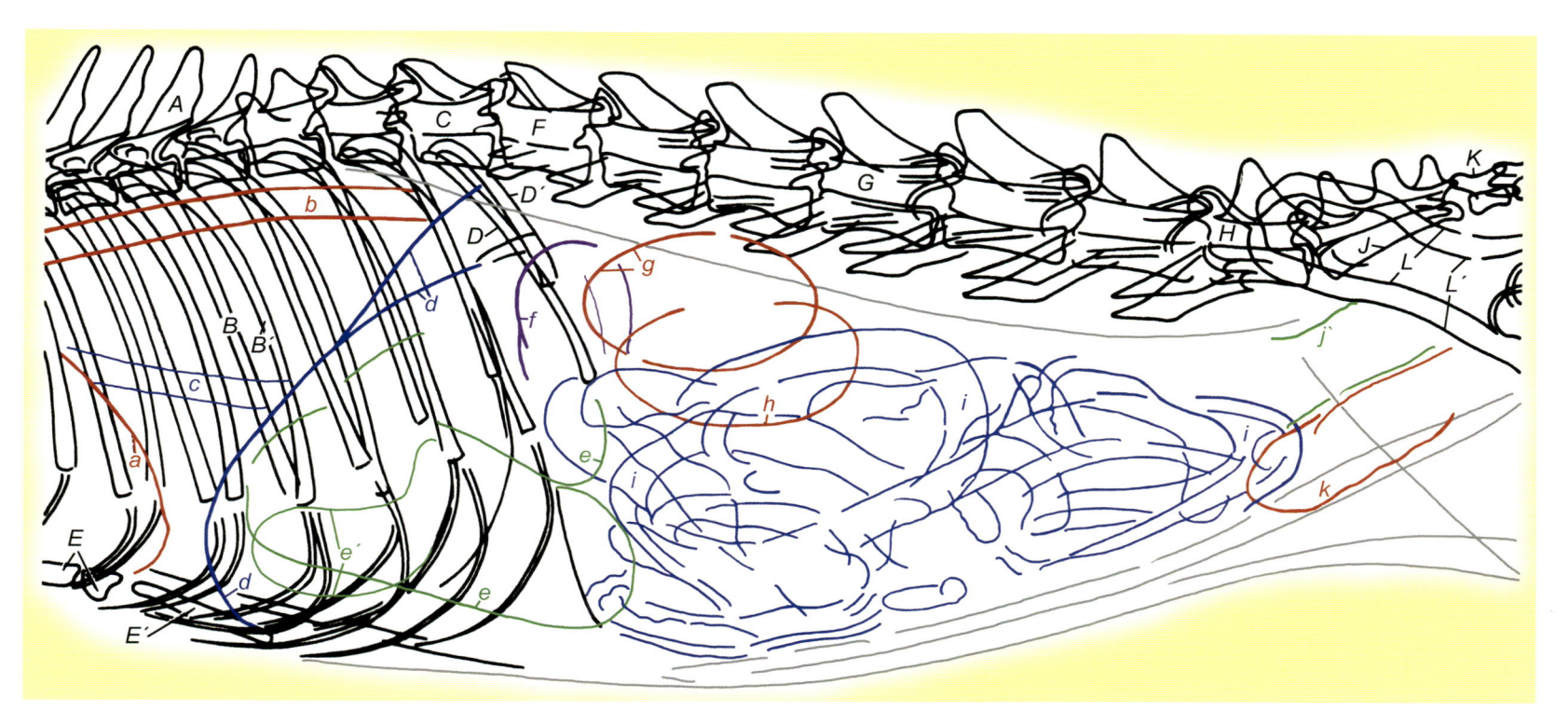

6.7 Cholezystographie, Gallenblase – Cholecystography, gallbladder ■ latero-lateral

A T IX

B Os costale IX, B´ plattenfern – *next to the tube*

C T XIII

D Os costale XIII, D´ plattenfern – *next to the tube*

E Sternebrae

E´ Proc. xiphoideus

F L I

G L IV

H L VII

J Os sacrum

K Co I

L Os ilium, L´ plattenfern – *next to the tube*

a Cor

b Aorta thoracica

c Vena cava caudalis

d Diaphragma

e Hepar

e´ Vesica fellea

f Ventriculus

g Ren dexter

h Ren sinister

i Intestinum (zum Teil gashaltig – *partly filled with gas*)

j Colon descendens

k Vesica urinaria

105

6 Abdomen – Abdomen

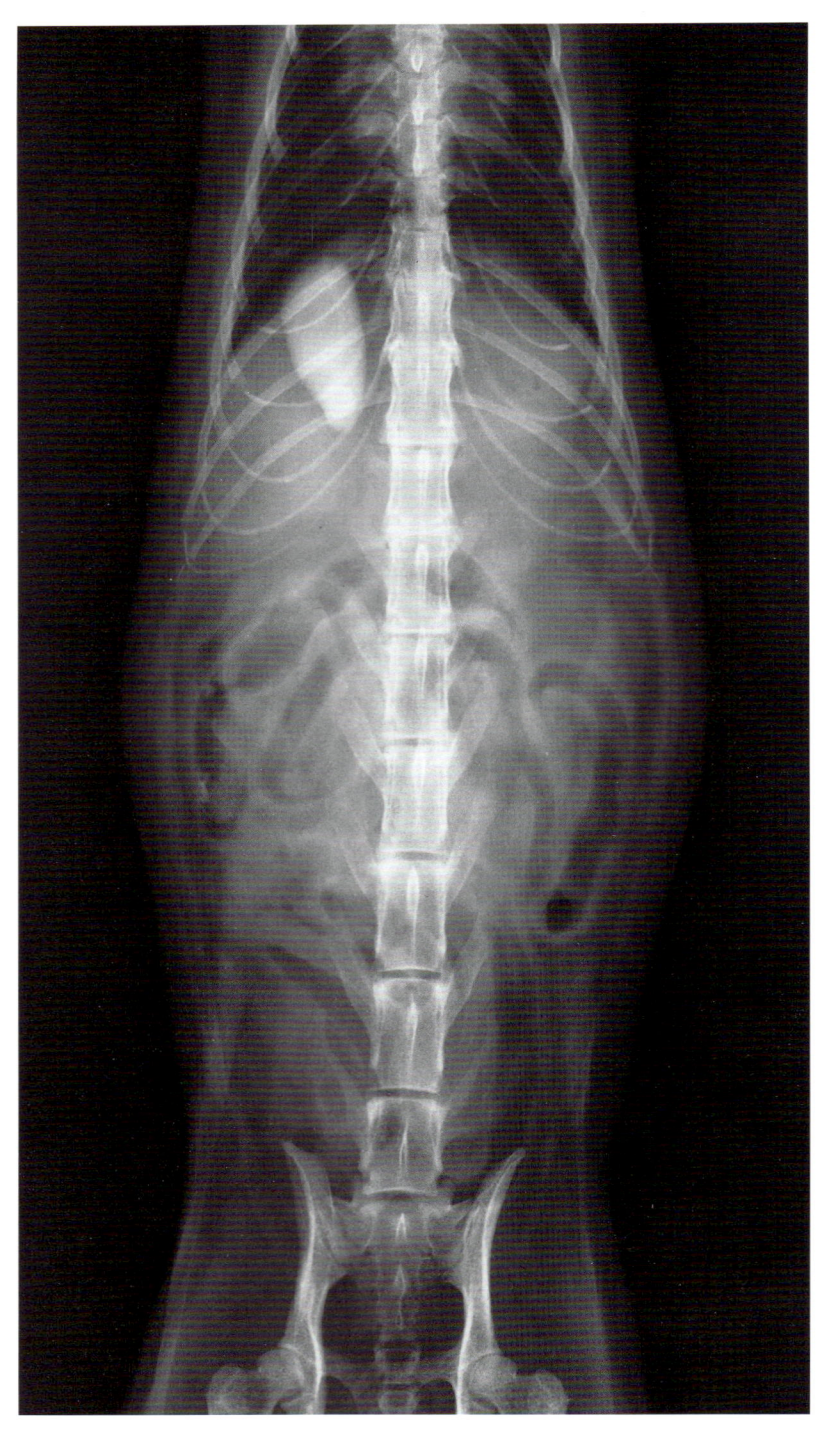

**Abb. 6.8 Gallenblasen-Darstellung,
ventro-dorsal**
(Biloptin®, Schering),
Katze
(Verkleinerung von 15 × 40 cm)

*Fig. 6.8 Gallbladder-contrast,
ventro-dorsal*
(Biloptin®, Schering),
Cat
(reduced from 15 × 40 cm)

■ Ziel
Übersichtsaufnahme der Bauchorgane, mit Kontrastdarstellung der Gallenblase.

■ Zentralstrahl
Senkrecht zur Kassette, auf die Medianebene, in Höhe des 3. Lendenwirbels.

■ Beachte
Lagerung kann durch Schaumgummikeile erreicht werden. Beckengliedmaße nach kaudal strecken.
Seitenbestimmung nicht vergessen!

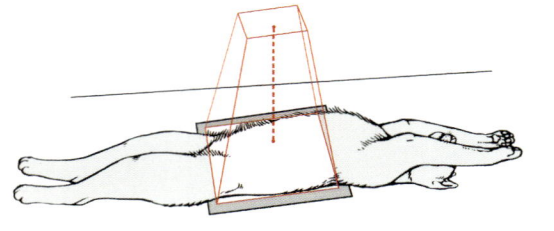

Abb. 6.8 Lagerung zur Aufnahme des Abdomens. Ventro-dorsal.

Diese Untersuchungstechnik wurde nahezu vollständig durch die Sonographie ersetzt.

*Fig. 6.8 Positioning of the abdomen.
Ventro-dorsal.*

This technique was replaced nearly completely by sonography.

■ *Objective*
To obtain a ventro-dorsal contrast radiographic study of the gallbladder.

■ *Central ray of the primary beam*
Direct the x-ray beam perpendicular to the cassette, with the central ray centered on the median plane, at the level of L 3.

■ *Notice*
Positioning can be supported by foam rubber wedges, stretch pelvic limbs caudally.
Do not forget the L/R mark!

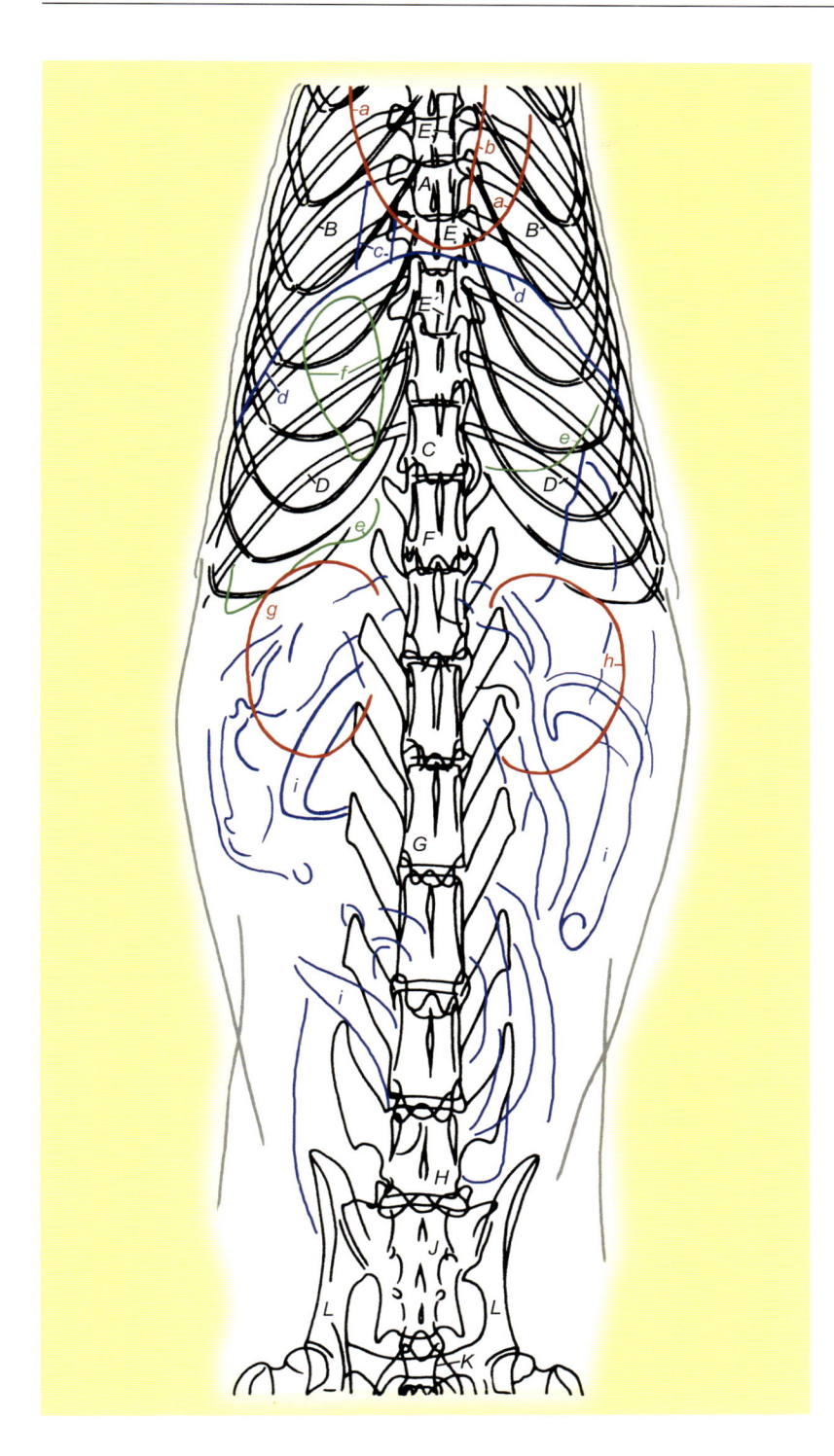

6.8 Cholezystographie, Gallenblase – Cholecystography, gallbladder ■ ventro-dorsal

A   T IX
B   Os costale IX
C   T XIII
D   Os costale XIII
E   Sternebrae
E´ Proc. xiphoideus
F   L I
G   L IV
H   L VII
J   Os sacrum
K   Co I
L   Os ilium

a   Cor
b   Aorta thoracica
c   Vena cava caudalis
d   Diaphragma
e   Hepar
f   Vesica fellea
g   Ren dexter
h   Ren sinister
i   Intestinum (zum Teil gashaltig – *partly filled with gas*)

107

Allgemeines zur Ausscheidungsurographie (Pyelozystographie)

Damit wird die Kontrastdarstellung der Nieren und ableitenden Harnwege nach intravenöser Verabreichung eines körperwarmen, wasserlöslichen jodhaltigen (= schattengebenden) Kontrastmittels bezeichnet. Es können dadurch nicht nur morphologische Veränderungen des Nierenparenchyms und des Nierenbeckens, der Harnleiter oder Harnblase erkannt, sondern aufgrund der Ausscheidungsgeschwindigkeit des Kontrastmittels auch eine grobe Funktionsprüfung der Nieren abgelesen werden.

Vorbereitung: Für das Tier ist ein 12- bis 24-stündiger Futterentzug angezeigt; Dürsten ist zu vermeiden.

Vor der Untersuchung sind Abdomen-Leeraufnahmen in 2 Ebenen anzufertigen, die einen Überblick über den Magen-Darm-Trakt und den Harntrakt geben. Gegebenenfalls ist ein Reinigungseinlauf spätestens 1 Stunde vor der Kontrastuntersuchung zur vollständigen Entleerung des Dickdarmes durchzuführen. Die Harnblase sollte weitgehend leer sein. Notfallpatienten dürfen erst nach Stabilisierung des Kreislaufes und des Flüssigkeitshaushaltes einer Kontrastuntersuchung unterzogen werden. Besondere Vorsicht ist bei hochgradiger Exsikkose geboten, eine Kontrastuntersuchung ist hier kontraindiziert.

Kontrastmittel: Bestens verträglich sind nichtionische wasserlösliche und jodhaltige Röntgenkontrastmittel (z.B. Iobitridol – Xenetix®, Guerbet; Iodixanol – Visipaque®, Nycomed; Iohexol – Omnipaque®, Schering; Iomeprol – Iomeron®, Gerot; Iopentol – Imagopaque®, Nycomed; Iopromid – Ultravist®, Schering; Ioversol – Optiray®, Mallinckrodt; Jopamidol – Jopamiro®, Gerot), auch ionische Zubereitungen sind möglich (Amidotrizoat – Urografin 76%®, Schering; Ioxaglinsäure – Hexabrix®, Guerbet; Ioxitalat und Meglumin – Telebrix®, Guerbet; Mediniumgluconat – Rayvist®, Schering; Megluminjodamid – Uromiro®, Gerot).

Dosis und Applikation: Für eine ausreichend beurteilbare Kontrastierung des Nierenparenchyms, des Nierenbeckens und der Harnleiter sind mindestens 500 mg Jod pro kg Körpermasse intravenös zu applizieren. Bei einem durchschnittlichen Jodgehalt von 250 bis 350 mg Jod pro ml Lösung entspricht dies zumindest 1,5 bis 2 ml Lösung pro kg Körpermasse.

Als applizierbare Obergrenze sind 1000 mg Jod pro kg Körpermasse anzusehen.

Bei der nicht zu schnellen intravenösen Applikation ist auf Zeichen einer Kontrastmittelunverträglichkeit zu achten, welche sich in geringem Grade durch Würgen, Schlecken oder auch Erbrechen des Tieres äußern. Höhergradige Unverträglichkeit mit Kollapszeichen ist extrem selten zu beobachten.

Untersuchungstechnik: Unmittelbar nach Beendigung der Applikation ist eine Aufnahme in Rückenlage zur Beurteilung der Anreicherung des Kontrastmittels in den Nieren (Parenchymphase) durchzuführen.

Nach weiteren 5 Minuten sind Aufnahmen in ventro-dorsaler und seitlicher Projektion anzuschließen, die bereits deutlich markierte Recessus collaterales und ein schmales Nierenbecken sowie die schlanken abführenden Ureteren zeigen (Pyelographiephase). Die früher geübte Manipulation mit Kompression des Bauches und damit der Ureteren zum Rückstau des Kontrastmittels für eine einwandfreie Nierenbeckendarstellung ist nicht mehr erforderlich. Die Ureteren stellen sich aufgrund der Ureterperistaltik nicht immer im gesamten Verlauf dar, eine Durchleuchtung ist daher empfehlenswert. Bei fraglichem ektopischem Ureter sind durchleuchtungsgezielte Aufnahmen der Ureterenmündung in der Frühphase der Ausscheidung angezeigt.

Nach weiteren 5–10 Minuten ist ein weiteres Bilderpaar zur Dokumentation des Höhepunktes der Kontrastmittelausscheidung anzufertigen, die zunehmende Markierung der Harnblase erlaubt deren Beurteilung. Die Schattendichte der Nieren nimmt nunmehr kontinuierlich ab. Nach etwa 20–30 Minuten ist die Ausscheidung des Kontrastmittels über die Nieren erfolgt, die Harnblase ist vollständig gefüllt. Bei Nierenschädigung verzögert sich die Kontrastmittelausscheidung über einige Stunden; bei offensichtlichem Nierenschaden, kenntlich an erhöhtem Creatinin und Harnstoff, sollte die Indikation zur Untersuchung streng gestellt und auf andere Verfahren wie die Ultraschalluntersuchung verwiesen werden.

Retrograde Zystographie: Die Untersuchung erfordert eine geeignete Ruhigstellung (Anästhesie). Der sterilisierte Katheter wird nach lokaler Reinigung in die Harnblase eingeführt, und Harn wird so lange abgelassen, bis die Harnblase nur noch geringgradig gefüllt ist. Gegen mögliche Schmerzen und Krämpfe der Harnblase kann eine lokale Gabe von Lidocain empfehlenswert sein.

Positivkontrast: 3–5 ml eines jodhaltigen Kontrastmittels (s.o.) werden appliziert.

Negativkontrast: 10–20 ml Raumluft werden insuffliert.

Doppelkontrast-Verfahren: 1 ml positives Kontrastmittel, danach etwa 10–15 ml Luft werden appliziert.

Bei Läsionen der Harnblase sollte unbedingt positives Kontrastmittel verwendet werden, ein etwaiger Austritt von Luft kann sehr leicht übersehen werden.

General remarks on excretory urography (pyelocystography)

Excretory urography is a contrast study of the kidneys, ureters, and urinary bladder after an intravenous injection of a water-soluble, iodinated (opacifying) medium at body temperature. It is not only a means of diagnosing morphological alterations, but is also a method to assess, to some degree, renal function.

Preparation of the patient: Withhold food for 12–24 hours, but do not withhold water! Obtain abdominal radiographs in two planes prior to the examination in order to gain a survey on the gastrointestinal and the urinary tract. If necessary, administer cleansing enemas at least one hour before the examination. The urinary bladder should be empty. In emergency cases, blood and fluid balance should be stabilized before contrast study. Hydration and renal blood chemistry should be assessed, because dehydration is a contraindication for this study.

Contrast media: Non-ionic, water-soluble and iodinated contrast media (e.g. iobitridol – Xenetix®, Guerbet; iodixanol – Visipaque®, Nycomed; iohexol – Omnipaque®, Schering; iomeprol – Iomeron®, Gerot; iopentol – Imagopaque®, Nycomed; iopromide – Ultravist®, Schering; ioversol – Optiray®, Mallinckrodt; jopamidol – Jopamiro®, Gerot) are well tolerated, but ionic preparations (amidotrizoate – Urografin 76%®, Schering; ioxaglic acid – Hexabrix®, Guerbet; meglumine ioxitalamate – Telebrix®, Guerbet; ioglicate – Rayvist®, Schering; iodamide – Uromiro®, Gerot) can also be used.

Dosage and administration: The warmed contrast medium is injected intravenously at a dosage of approximately 500 mg iodine/kg body weight to gain sufficient opacification of the renal parenchyma, renal pelvis, and ureters. The rule of thumb dose is 1.5–2 ml/kg body weight, if the contrast medium contains an iodine dose of 250–350 mg/ml. A maximum iodine dose of 1000 mg/kg body weight has been used. Although less effective, a subcutaneous injection is possible, with radiographs taken 15 minutes after injection. During the intravenous injection watch out for systemic shock reactions, such as choking, licking or vomiting. Severe adverse reactions such as collapse are very rare.

Technique: Obtain abdominal radiographs in the following sequence: ventrodorsal view just after injection of the contrast medium to image the renal parenchyma, nephrogram phase); ventrodorsal and lateral views 5 minutes later (to image the renal pelvis, pelvic recesses, and ureters, pyelographic phase); and additional radiographs in two planes 5–10 minutes later (to image fading of the renal parenchyma and pelvis, and opacification of the urinary bladder). The diameter of the ureter will vary along its course due to peristaltic movement of the contrast medium. If an ectopic ureter is suspected, fluoroscopy may better be used to better visualize the distal ureters and the ureterovesicular junctions. Another set of radiographs 20–30 minutes after injection should show most or all of the contrast medium within the urinary bladder.

The formerly used abdominal compression technique, which assisted in better visualization of the renal collecting system and proximal ureters by delaying clearance of the contrast medium, is no longer recommended.

In case of impaired renal function, the excretory urogram may be prolonged by as much as several hours. In patients with severe renal compromise as indicated by increased serum creatinine and blood urea concentrations, excretory urography is contraindicated, and should be replaced by other diagnostic techniques such as sonography.

Retrograde contrast cystography: This examination requires that the patient be heavily sedated or placed under general anesthesia. Only a sterilized catheter should be used, and the genitalia should be thoroughly cleaned before the bladder is catheterized. To reduce bladder pain and spasm during cystography, lidocaine instillation may be recommended. The catheter is passed through the urethra into the urinary bladder, and urine is removed until the bladder is only slightly filled.

Positive-contrast examination: 3–5 ml of a non-iodinated contrast medium is injected through the catheter into the urinary bladder.

Negative-contrast examination: 10–20 ml of room air (or CO_2) is carefully injected. If resistance is encountered, do not forcefully inject the gas. In rare cases of chronic cystitis (non-elastic bladder wall), the forceful injection of air has resulted in air emboli in the bloodstream, which can be fatal. Note: In the unlikely event of emboli formation, CO_2 has the advantage of being much more soluble in blood than room air.

Double-contrast examination: 1 ml of positive-contrast medium, followed by approximately 10–15 ml room air is injected through the catheter.

If perforation of the urinary bladder is suspected, a positive-contrast procedure only is recommended.

6 Abdomen – Abdomen

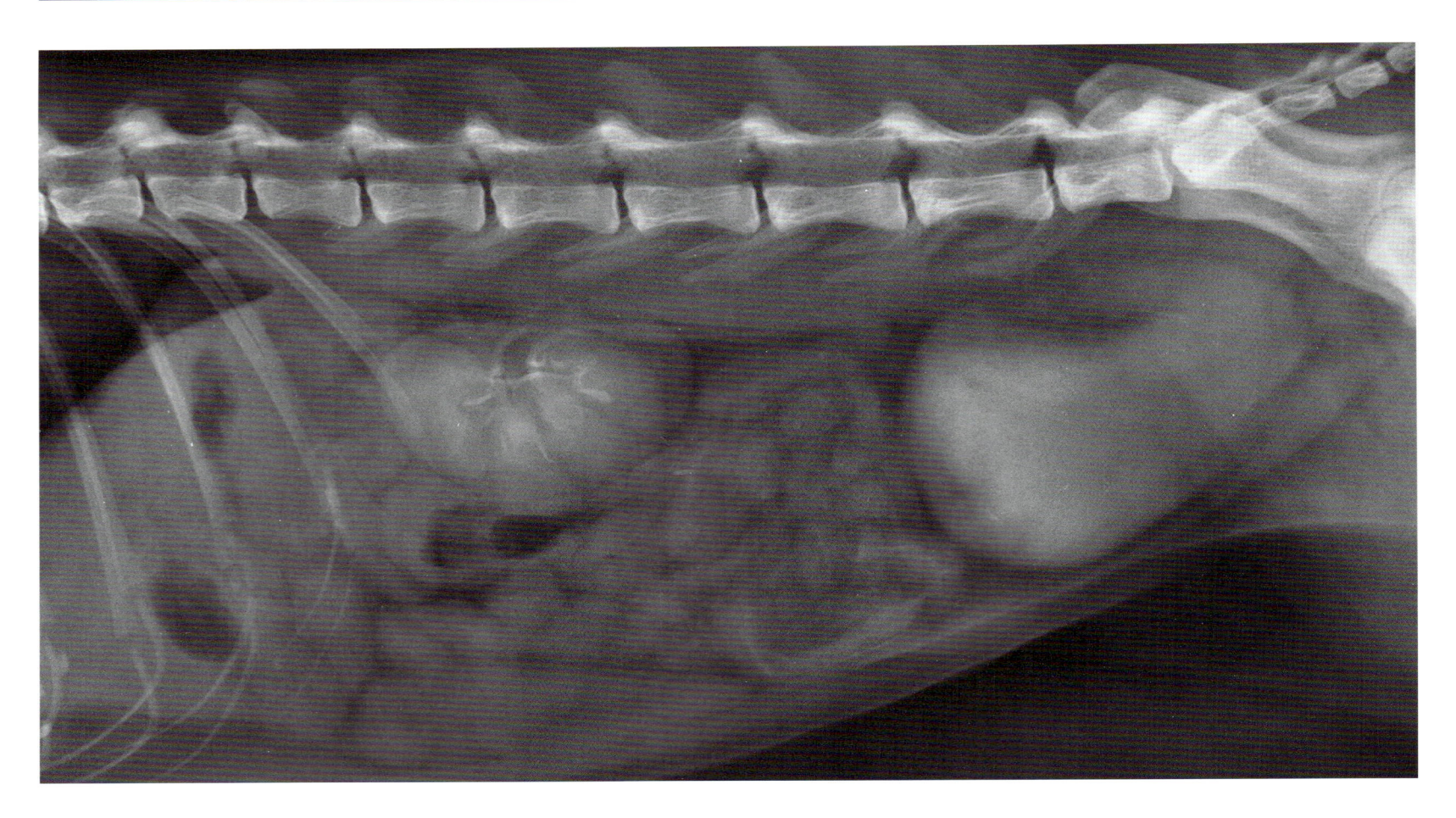

Abb. 6.9 Pyelographie, liegend, latero-lateral
(Urografin 76 %, Schering),
Katze
(Verkleinerung von 24 × 30 cm)

Fig. 6.9 Pyelography, recumbent, latero-lateral
(Urografin 76%, Schering),
Cat
(reduced from 24 × 30 cm)

■ **Ziel**
Kontrastaufnahme der Nieren und des Harnleiters (Aufnahme speziell der Nierenregion, der Ureteren und der Harnblase).

■ **Zentralstrahl**
Senkrecht zur Kassette, auf die Regio abdominis lateralis in Höhe des 4. Lendenwirbels.

■ **Beachte**
Die Medianebene soll parallel zur Kassette gelagert sein, bei fettleibigen Katzen kann dies durch Unterlegen eines Schaumgummikeils erreicht werden; die Beckengliedmaßen nach kaudal strecken.

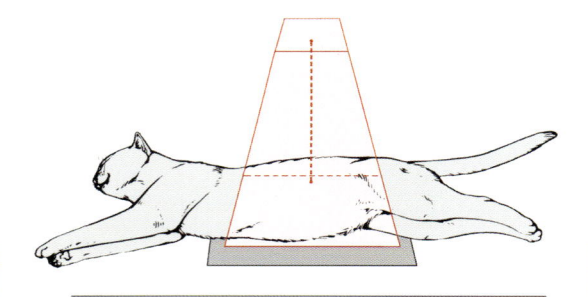

Abb. 6.9 Lagerung zur Aufnahme des Abdomens. Latero-lateral.

Fig. 6.9 Positioning of the abdomen. Latero-lateral.

■ *Objective*
To obtain a lateral contrast study of the kidneys, ureters, and urinary bladder.

■ *Central ray of the primary beam*
Direct the x-ray beam perpendicular to the cassette, with the central ray centered on the lateral abdomen, at the level of L4.

■ *Notice*
Align the cassette parallel to the median plane, use a foam rubber wedge in obese patients, stretch the pelvic limbs caudally.

6.9 Pyelographie – Pyelography ■ latero-lateral

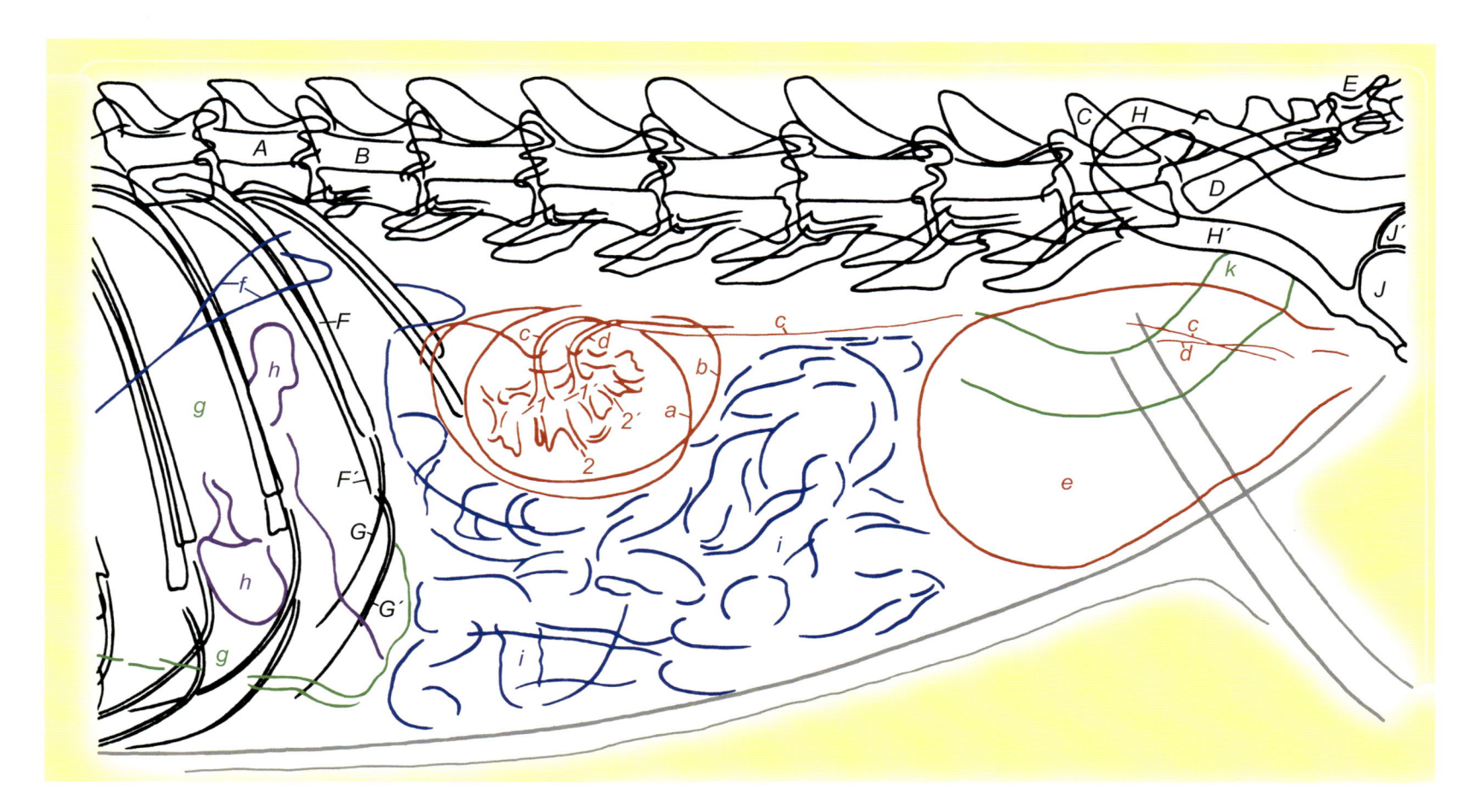

A   T XIII

B   L I

C   L VII

D   Os sacrum

E   Co I

F   Os costale XII, F´ plattenfern – *next to the tube*

G   Cartilago costalis XII, G´ plattenfern – *next to the tube*

H   Os ilium, H´ plattenfern – *next to the tube*

J   Caput ossis femoris, J´ plattenfern – *next to the tube*

a   Ren dexter
   1   Pelvis renalis
   2   Recessus pelvis

b   Ren sinister
   1´ Pelvis renalis
   2´ Recessus pelvis

c   Ureter dexter

d   Ureter sinister

e   Vesica urinaria

f   Diaphragma

g   Hepar

h   Ventriculus (zum Teil gashaltig – *partly filled with gas*)

i   Intestinum tenue

k   Colon descendens

111

6 Abdomen – Abdomen

Abb. 6.10 Pyelographie, liegend, ventro-dorsal
(Urografin 76%, Schering),
Katze
(Verkleinerung von 24 × 30 cm)

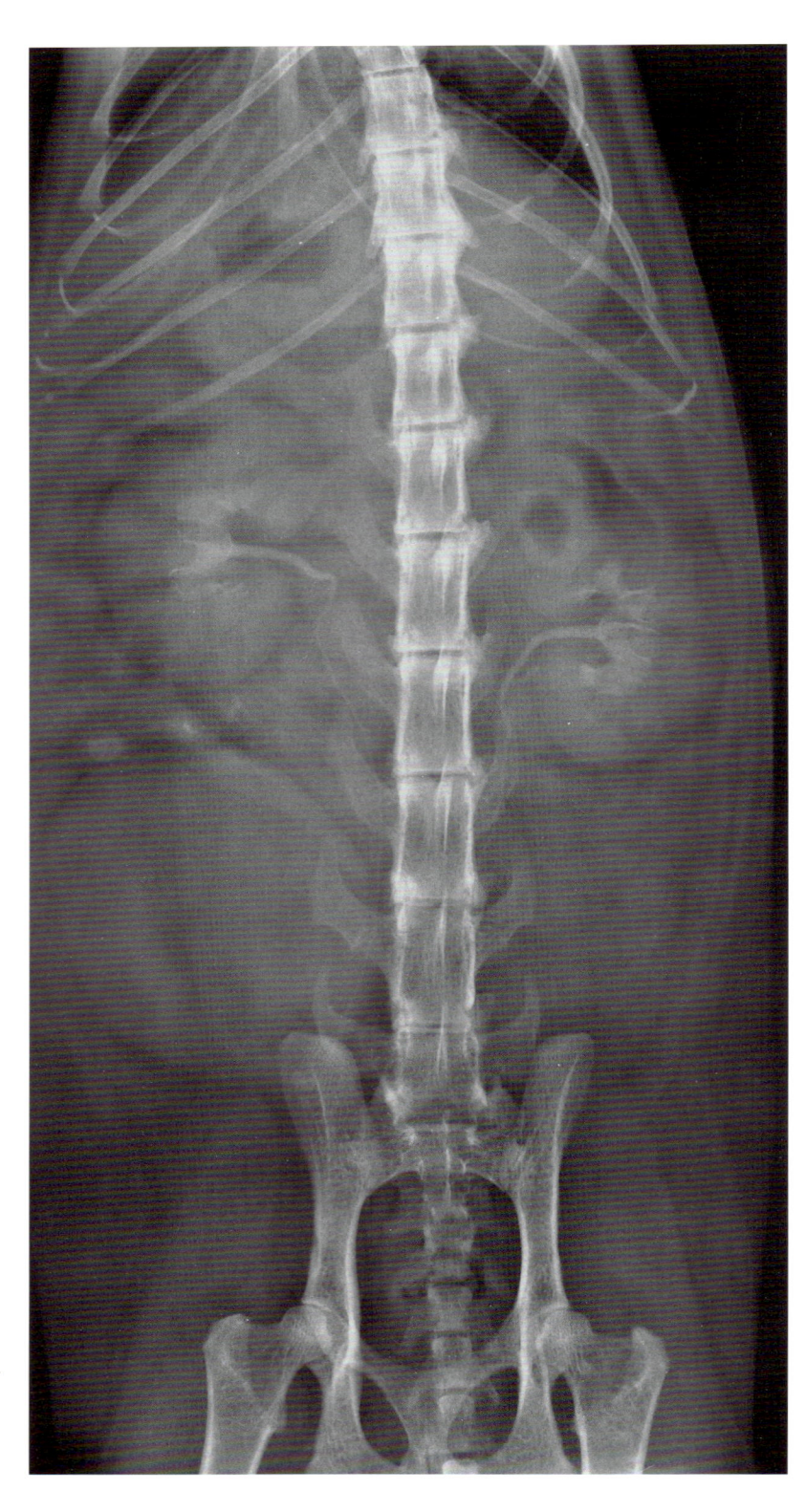

Fig. 6.10 Pyelography, recumbent, ventro-dorsal
*(Urografin 76%, Schering),
Cat
(reduced from 24 × 30 cm)*

■ **Ziel**
Kontrastaufnahme der Nieren und des Harnleiters (Aufnahme speziell der Nierenregion, der Ureteren und der Harnblase).

■ **Zentralstrahl**
Senkrecht zur Kassette, auf die Medianebene, in Höhe des 4. Lendenwirbels.

■ **Beachte**
Die Medianebene soll parallel zur Kassette gelagert sein, dies kann durch Unterlegen eines Schaumgummikeils erreicht werden; die Beckengliedmaßen nach kaudal strecken.

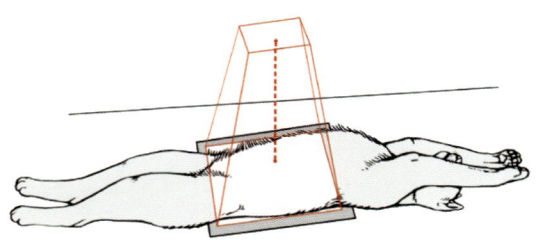

Abb. 6.10 Lagerung zur Aufnahme des Abdomens. Ventro-dorsal.

Fig. 6.10 Positioning of the abdomen. Ventro-dorsal.

■ *Objective*
To obtain a ventro-dorsal contrast study of the kidneys, ureters, and urinary bladder.

■ *Central ray of the primary beam*
Direct the x-ray beam perpendicular to the cassette, with the central ray centered on the median plane, at the level of L 4.

■ *Notice*
Align the cassette perpendicular to the median plane, use a foam rubber wedge, stretch pelvic limbs caudally.

6.10 Pyelographie – Pyelography ■ ventro-dorsal

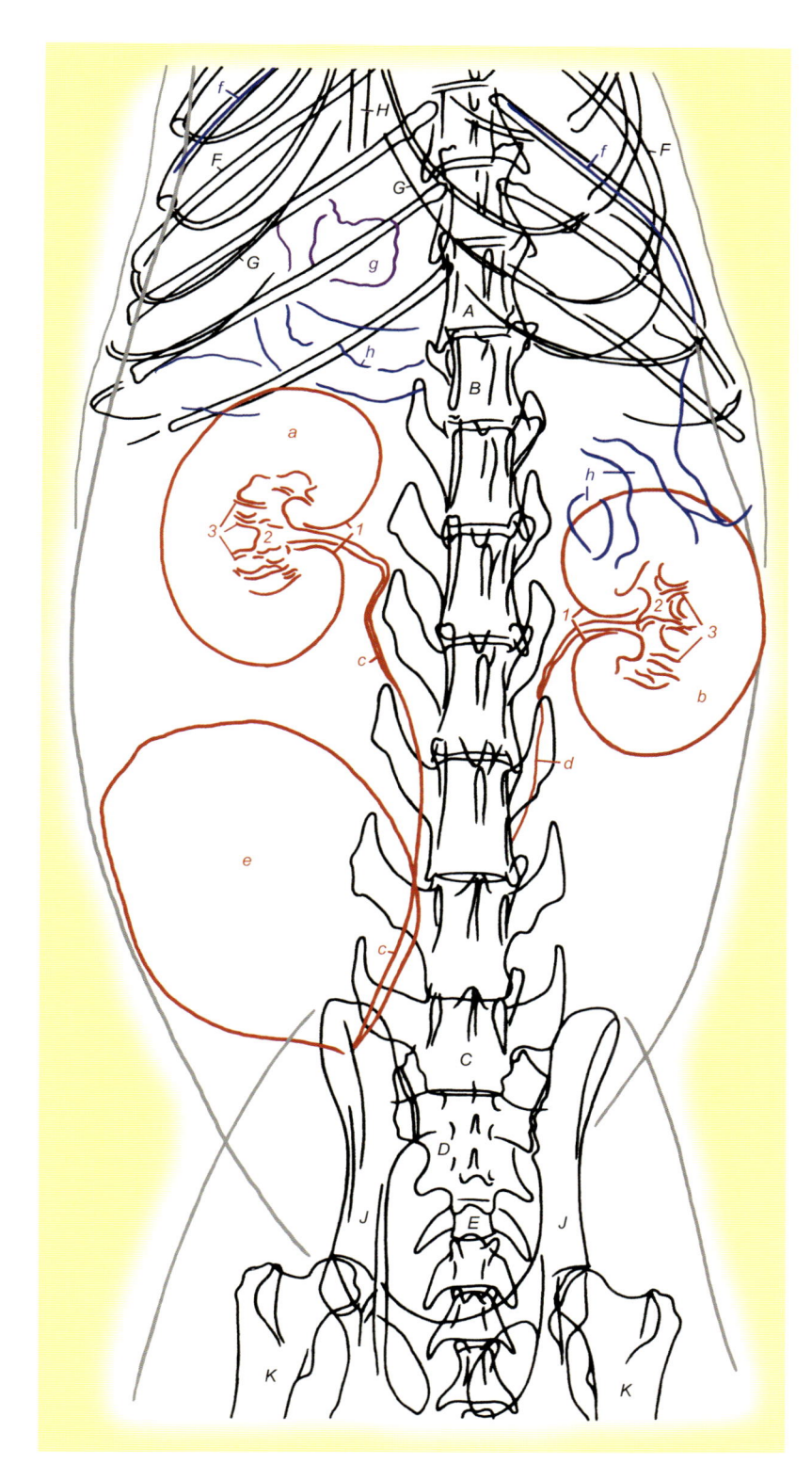

A T XIII

B L I

C L VII

D Os sacrum

E Co I

F Os costale X

G Cartilago costalis X

H Processus xiphoideus

J Os ilium

K Os femoris

a **Ren dexter**
   1   Hilus renalis
   2   Pelvis renalis
   3   Recessus pelvis

b **Ren sinister**
   1   Hilus renalis
   2   Pelvis renalis
   3   Recessus pelvis

c Ureter dexter

d Ureter sinister

e Vesica urinaria

f Diaphragma

g Ventriculus

h Intestinum (zum Teil gashaltig – *partly filled with gas*)

6 Abdomen – Abdomen

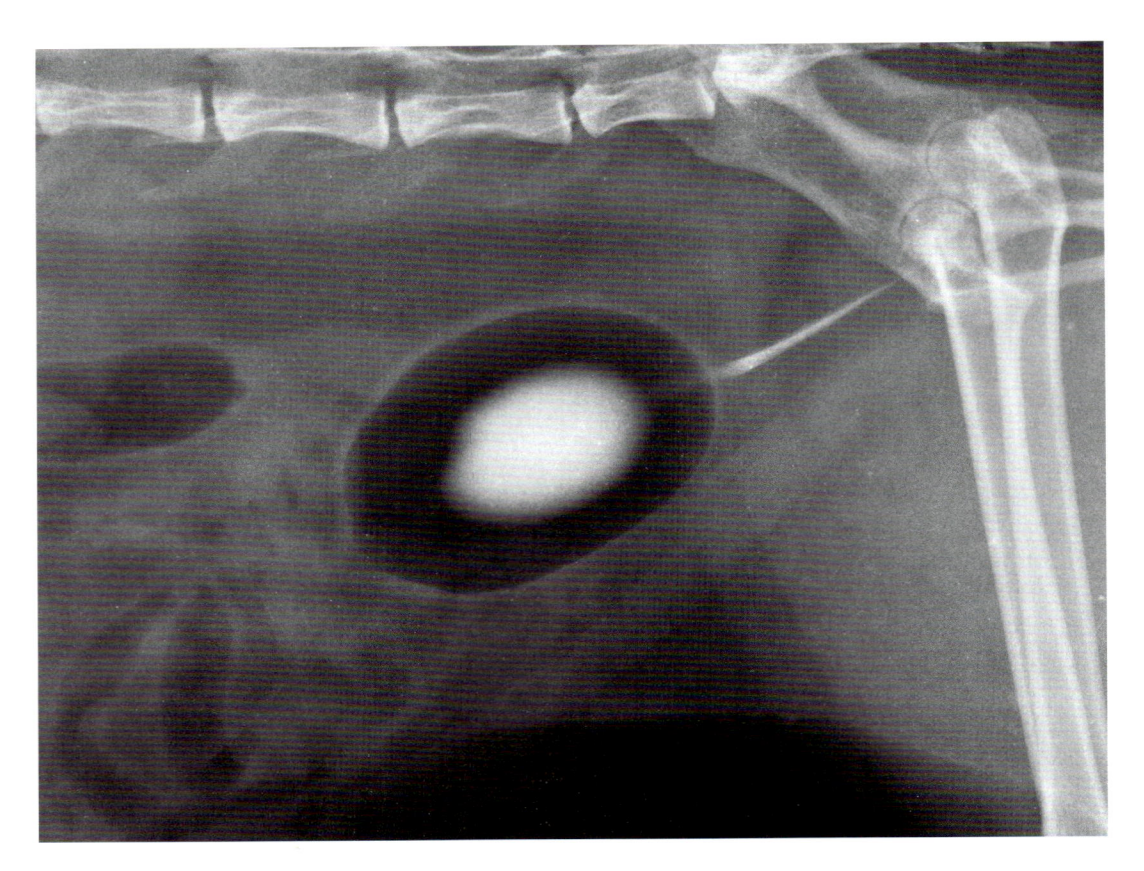

Abb. 6.11 Harnblase, Negativ- und Positiv-Kontrast, liegend, latero-lateral
(Luft und Kaliumjodid 10%ig),
Katze
(Ausschnitt aus 18 × 24 cm)

Fig. 6.11 Urinary bladder, double-contrast, recumbent, latero-lateral
(air and 10% potassium iodide),
Cat
(section of 18 × 24 cm)

■ **Ziel**
Positiv-negativ-Kontrast-Darstellung der Harnblase.

■ **Zentralstrahl**
Senkrecht zur Kassette, auf die Regio abdominis lateralis in Höhe des 6. Lendenwirbels.

■ *Objective*
To obtain a double-contrast (positive & negative) radiograph of the urinary bladder.

■ *Central ray of the primary beam*
Direct the central ray of the x-ray beam perpendicular to the cassette, centered on the lateral abdominal region, at the level of L6.

■ **Beachte**
Symmetrische Streckung der Schultergliedmaßen nach vorn und der Beckengliedmaßen nach hinten.

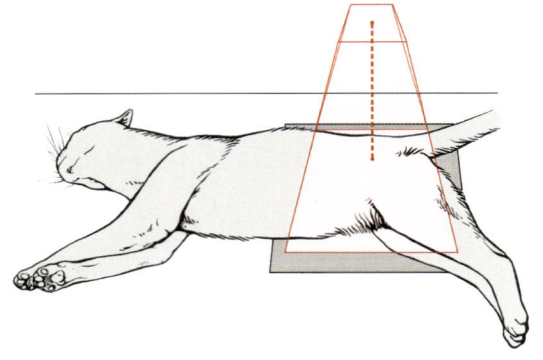

Abb. 6.11 Lagerung zur Aufnahme des Abdomens/der Harnblase. Latero-lateral.

Fig. 6.11 Positioning of the abdomen/survey radiograph of the urinary bladder. Latero-lateral.

■ *Notice*
Symmetric extension of the thoracic limbs cranially and the pelvic limbs caudally.

6.11 Zystographie – Cystography ■ latero-lateral

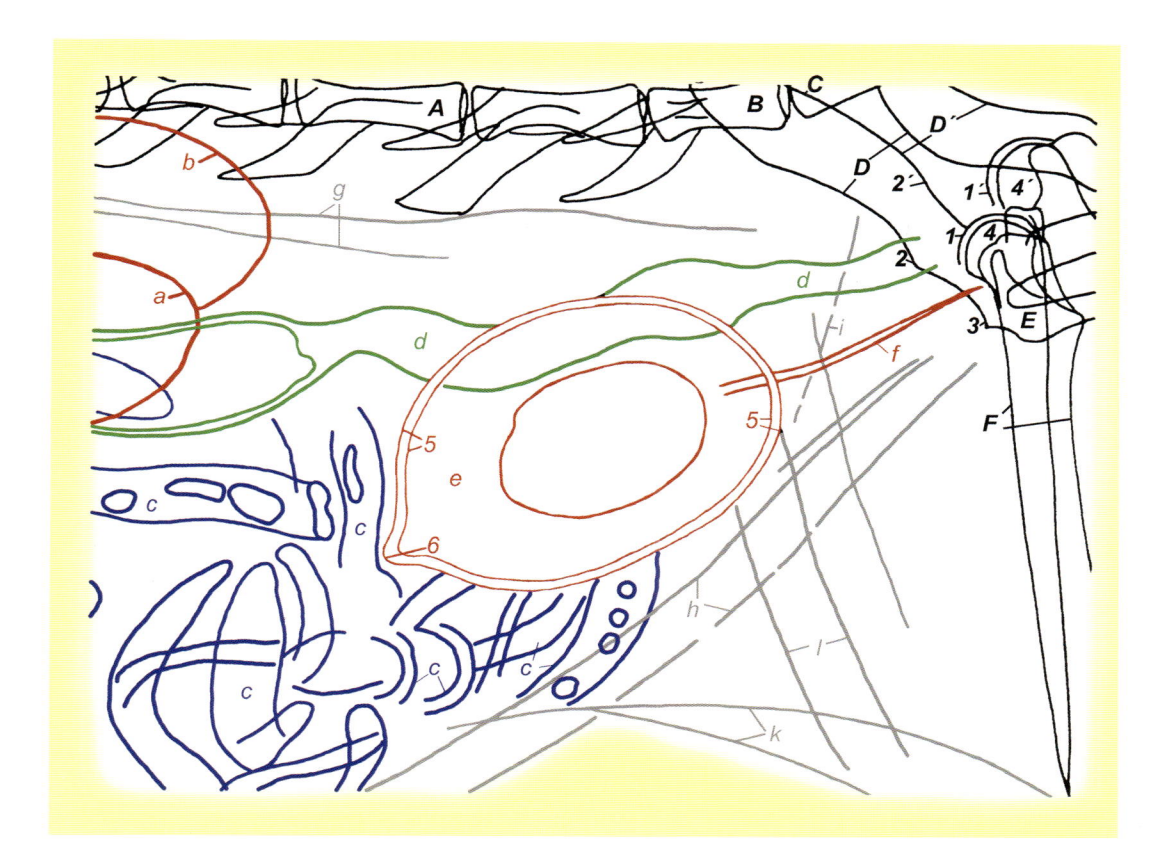

A L V

B L VII

C Os sacrum

D Os ilium, D´ plattenfern – *next to the tube*

E Os pubis
    1 Acetabulum, 1´ plattenfern – *next to the tube*
    2 Eminentia iliopubica, 2´ plattenfern – *next to the tube*
    3 Pecten ossis pubis

F Os femoris
    4 Caput ossis femoris, 4´ plattenfern – *next to the tube*

a Ren dexter

b Ren sinister

c Intestinum tenue (zum Teil mit Gas gefüllt – *partly filled with gas*)

d Colon descendens (zum Teil mit Gas gefüllt – *partly filled with gas*)

e Vesica urinaria
    5 Harnblasenwand – *wall of the urinary bladder*
    6 Urachusnabel – *Umbilicus of the urachus*

f Urethra

g innere Lendenmuskulatur, ventrale Begrenzung – *inner lumbar muscles, ventral border*

h ventrale Bauchwand – *ventral abdominal wall*

i Musculus transversus abdominis

k Plica lateris, Kniefalte – *fold of the flank*

l kraniale Kontur des Oberschenkels – *cranial outline of the thigh*

Literatur – References

Adin, C.A., E.J. Herrgesell, T.G. Nyland, J.M. Hughes, C.R. Gregory, A.E. Kyles, L.D. Cowgill and G.V. Ling (2003): Antegrade pyelography for suspected ureteral obstruction in cats: 11 cases (1995–2001). J. Am. Vet. Med. Assoc. **222**, 1576–1581.

Agut, A., J. Murciano, M.A. Sanchez-Valverde, F.G. Laredo and M.C. Tovar (1999): Comparison of different doses of iohexol with amidotrizoate for excretory urography in cats. Res. Vet. Sci. **67**, 73–82.

Ahlberg, N.E., Hansson, K., Svensson, L. and K. Iwarsson (1989): Radiographic heart-volume estimation in normal cats. Vet. Rad. **30**, 253–260.

Armbrust, L.J., D.S. Biller and J.J. Hoskinson (2000): Case examples demonstrating the clinical utility of obtaining both right and left lateral abdominal radiographs in small animals. J. Am. Anim. Hosp. Assoc. **36**, 531–536.

Armbrust, L.J., D.S. Biller and J.J. Hoskinson (2000): Compression radiography: an old technique revisited. J. Am. Anim. Hosp. Assoc. **36**, 537–541.

Arnberg, J. and N.I. Heje (1993): Fabellae and popliteal sesamoid bones in cats. JSAP **34**, 5–8.

Brawner, W.R. and J.E. Bartels (1983): Contrast radiography of the digestive tract. Vet. Clin. North Am. **13**, 599–626.

Buchtala, V. und H.P. Jensen (1955): Die Probleme der zerebralen Angiographie. Fortschr. Röntgenstr. **82**, 76.

Carlisle, C.H. (1977): Radiographic anatomy of the cat gallbladder. JAVRS **18**, 170–172.

Carlisle, C.H. (1977): A comparison of technics for cholecystography in the cat. JAVRS **18**, 173–176.

Carlisle, C.H. and D.E. Thrall (1982): A comparison of normal feline thoracic radiographs made in dorsal versus ventral recumbency. Vet. Rad. **23**, 3–9.

Eisner, E.R. (1998): Oral-dental radiographic examination technique. Vet. Clin. North Am. Small Anim. Pract. **28**, 1063–1087.

Farrow, C.S. (1974): Retrograde urography in the cat. VM/SAC **69**, 435–437.

Farrow, C.S. (1984): The radiology of aging: its clinical applications. Comp. Cont. Ed. **6**, 1114.

Farrow, C.S. and R.E. Bach (1980): Gastrointestinal contrast examination in the cat. Fel. Pract. **10**, 20–25.

Forterre, F., B. Gutmannsbauer, W. Schmahl and U. Matis (1998): CT myelography for diagnosis of brachial plexus avulsion in small animals. Tierärztl. Prax. **26**, 322–329.

Garosi, L.S., R. Dennis and T. Schwarz (2003): Review of diagnostic imaging of ear diseases in the dog and cat. Vet. Radiol. Ultrasound **44**, 137–146.

Gracis, M. (1999): Radiographic study of the maxillary canine tooth of four mesaticephalic cats. J. Vet. Dent. **16**, 115–128.

Hamlin, R.L., Smetzer, D.L. and C.R. Smith (1963): Radiographic anatomy of the normal cat heart. JAVMA **43**, 957–961.

Hofer, P., N. Meisen, S. Bartholdi and B. Kaser-Hotz (1995): A new radiographic view of the feline tympanic bullae. Vet. Radiol. Ultrasound **36**, 14–15.

Horvath, A. (1983): Röntgenanatomische Untersuchungen zur postnatalen Entwicklung des Hintergliedmaßenskeletts der Hauskatze *(Felis cattus)*. München, Diss. med. vet.

Horvath, I. (1983): Röntgenanatomische Untersuchungen zur postnatalen Entwicklung des Vordergliedmaßenskeletts der Hauskatze *(Felis cattus)*. München, Diss. med. vet.

Hoskinson, J.J. and R.L. Tucker (2001): Diagnostic imaging of lameness in small animals. Vet. Clin. North Am. Small Anim. Pract. **31**, 165–180.

Jensen, H.-P. (1954): Die zerebrale Seriographie mit dem Gerät nach Buchtala. Ärzt. Wschr. **9**, 468.

Kealy, J.K. and H. McAllister (1981): Radiology refresher no. 17: the radiology of the mediastinum. J. Small Anim. Pract. **22**, 717–729.

Kobara-Mates, M., J.A. Logemann, C. Larson and P.J. Kahrilas (1995): Physiology of oropharyngeal swallow in the cat: a videofluoroscopic and electromyographic study. Am. J. Physiol. **268**, 232–241.

Lamb, C.R., S. Richbell and P. Mantis (2003): Radiographic signs in cats with nasal disease. J. Feline Med. Surg. **5**, 227–235.

LeCouteur, R.A. (2003): Spinal cord disorders. J. Feline Med. Surg. **5**, 121–131.

Lommer, M.J. and F.J. Verstraete (2001): Radiographic patterns of periodontitis in cats: 147 cases (1998–1999). J. Am. Vet. Med. Assoc. **218**, 230–234.

Lora-Michiels, M., D.S. Biller, D. Olsen, J.J. Hoskinson, S.L. Kraft and J.C. Jones (2003): The accessory lung lobe in thoracic disease: a case series and anatomical review. J. Am. Anim. Hosp. Assoc. **39**, 452–458.

Lord, P.F. and W.J. Zontine (1985): Radiologic examination of the feline cardiovascular system. Vet. Clin. North Am. **7**, 291–307.

Morgan, J.P. (1977): The upper gastrointestinal tract in the cat: a protocol for contrast radiography. JAVRS **18**, 134–137.

Morgan, J.P. and S. Silverman (1993): Techniques of Veterinary Radiography. 5th Ed., Iowa State University Press/Ames.

Nykamp, S. and P. Scrivani (2001): Feline myelography. Vet. Radiol. Ultrasound **42**, 532–533.

Roos, H. (1989): Zur funktionellen und topographischen Anatomie der Schultergliedmaße der Hauskatze *(Felis silvestris f. catus)*. Habil.-Schrift, München.

Santilli, R.A. and G. Gerboni (2003): Diagnostic imaging of congenital porto-systemic shunts in dogs and cats: a review. Vet. J. **166**, 7–18.

Schwarz, L.A. and A.S. Tidwell (1999): Alternative imaging of the lung. Clin. Tech. Small Anim. Pract. **14**, 187–206.

Scrivani, P.V. (2000): Myelographic artifacts. Vet. Clin. North Am. Small Anim. Pract. **30**, 303–314.

Sis, R.F. and R. Getty (1968): Normal radiographic anatomy of the cat. Vet. Med. Small Anim. Clin. **63**, 475–492.

Smallwood, J.E., Shively, M.J., Rendano, V.T. and R.E. Habel (1985): A standardized nomenclature for radiographic projections used in veterinary medicine. Vet. Rad. **26**, 2–9.

Smith, R.N. (1968): Appearance of ossification centers in the kitten. J. Small Anim. Pract. **9**, 491–511.

Smith, R.N. (1969): Fusion of the ossification centers in the cat. J. Small Anim. Pract. **10**, 523–530.

Toal, R.L., J.M. Losonsky, D.B. Coulter and R. DeNovellis (1985): Influence of cardiac cycle on the radiographic appearance of the feline heart. Vet. Rad. **26**, 63–69.

Verstraete, F.J., P.H. Kass and C.H. Terpak (1998): Diagnostic value of full-mouth radiography in cats. Am. J. Vet. Res. **59**, 692–695.

Wheeler, S.J., D.G. Clayton Jones and J.A. Wright (1985): Myelography in the cat. J. Small Anim. Pract. **26**, 143.

Widmer, W.R. and W.E. Blevins (1991): Veterinary myelography: a review of contrast media, adverse effects, and technique. JAAHA **27**, 163.

White, R.N. and C.A. Burton (2001): Anatomy of the patent ductus venosus in the cat. J. Feline Med. Surg. **3**, 229–233.

Wise, M. (1982): Non-selective angiocardiography in the normal dog and cat. Vet. Rad. **23**, 144–151.

Umfassend, übersichtlich und praxisnah!

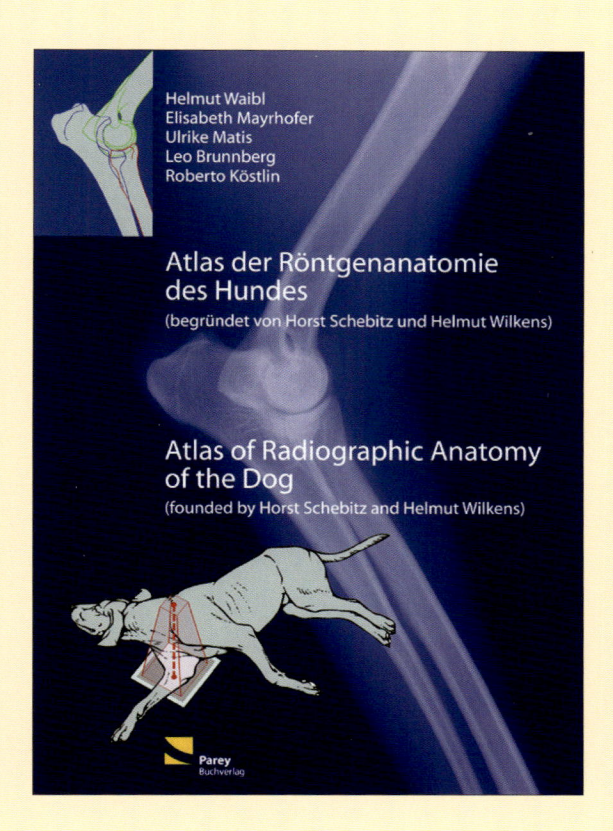

H. Waibl, E. Mayrhofer,
U. Matis, L. Brunnberg, R. Köstlin

Atlas der Röntgenanatomie des Hundes

Begründet von H. Schebitz und H. Wilkens
2003, 172 S., 243 Abb., 2 Tab., geb.
€ [D] 119,–
ISBN 3-8304-4064-2

Die Kenntnis der Röntgenanatomie ist die Basis zur Diagnose pathologischer Veränderungen beim Hund.

74 ausgesuchte Röntgenaufnahmen gesunder Hunde bilden die Grundlage für dieses in sechs topographische Kapitel (Kopf, Wirbelsäule, Schultergliedmaße, Beckengliedmaße, Thorax und Abdomen) geordnete Werk. Die farbige Darstellung und differenzierte Beschriftung der entsprechenden Röntgenskizzen verbessern die Übersichtlichkeit und erleichtern das Auffinden der gesuchten Strukturen.

Jeder Röntgendarstellung wurde auf der gleichen Seite ein entsprechender Lagerungsvorschlag mit beachtenswerten Ratschlägen hinzugefügt. Kurze Hinweise zur Lagerung und zur Belichtung von Röntgenaufnahmen sowie allgemeine Bemerkungen zu Kontrastdarstellungen ergänzen diesen Atlas. Farbige schematische Zeichnungen veranschaulichen die Entwicklung des Extremitätenskelettes in den ersten neun Monaten.

**MVS Medizinverlage Stuttgart
GmbH & Co. KG**
Postfach 30 05 04 • 70445 Stuttgart
Telefon 07 11 / 89 31-906
Fax 07 11 / 89 31-901

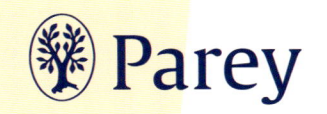

Parey